A BOOK

OF

MEDICAL DISCOURSES

IN TWO PARTS

A BOOK

OF

MEDICAL DISCOURSES

IN TWO PARTS

PART FIRST:

Creating of the cause, prevention, and cure of infantile bowel complaints, from birth to the close of the teething period, or till after the fifth year.

PART SECOND:

Containing misckllaneous information concerning the i.lfe and growth of beings; the beginning of woman-hood; also, the cause, prevention, ano cure of many of the most distressing complaints of women, and youth of both sexes.

BY

REBECCA CRUMPLER, M.D.

BOSTON:

CASHMAN, KEATING & CO., PRINTERS

FAYETTE COURT, 603 WASHINGTON ST.

1883

ISBN: 978-1-6673-0433-5 paperback
ISBN: 978-1-6673-0434-2 hardcover

DEDICATION

TO
MOTHERS, NURSES,

AND ALL WHO MAY DESIRE TO MITIGATE THE AFFLICTIONS OF THE HUMAN RACE

THIS BOOK

IS PRAYERFULLY OFFERED

CONTENTS

INTRODUCTION 9

PART FIRST. Creating of the Cause, Prevention, and Cure of Infantile Bowel Complaints, From Birth To the Close of the Teething Period, Or Till After the Fifth Year

I. How To Marry..15

II. The Present Modes of Washing and Dressing the New-Born...............17

III. Preparations for Confinement.......................................19

IV. The Better Mode of Washing the New-Born.............................21

V. Necessity of Agreeableand Soothing Surroundings......................25

VI. Nursing From the Breast Made Easy..................................27

VII. The Uselessness of "Baby Medicines" During the Month...............31

VIII. Dropping of the Navel Cord.......................................36

IX. Artificial Nursing...39

X. The Milk Fever..43

XI. Precautions After the Month – Proper and Improper Diet.............47

XII. General Treatment of Infants......................................52

XIII. Time for Weaning...56

XIV. SECTION I. Cholera infantum versus starvation.....................59

SECTION II. Symptoms of emptiness or starvation, which may lead to cholera..61

SECTION III. Cholera infantum – infantile cholera.....................62

SECTION IV. General treatment of cholera infantum, medical and domestic..65

XV.   The Causes and Preventionof Cholera Infantum 69

XVI.   Convenient Methods for Raising Infants without
        The Breast...72

XVII.   SECTION I. Teething made easy..79
        SECTION II. The order in which the teeth come 81

XVIII. Complications of Teething with Diseases 85

XIX.   General Remarks 91

PART SECOND

        Miscellaneous Information..105

NOTE 123

ERRATA..124

INTRODUCTION

I NOW present to the public a few thoughts in book form, trusting that they will be accepted on their merits alone. The following pages contain a few simple appeals to common sense, and are addressed to mothers, nurses, and women generally. All honor is due to a far-seeing legislation which has recognized the importance of fitting woman for the great and natural office of nurse, or doctress of medicine; for by it facilities are offered to each member of a community for the promotion of Christian enlightenment. By frequent visits through various parts of the United States, at all seasons of the year, as well as by quite an extensive opportunity while in the capacity of family nurse, and subsequent practitioner, I have become quite familiar with those ailments and diseases which afflict many infants from birth to the close of the teething period, or till after the fifth year of their age.

It may be well to state here that, having been reared by a kind aunt in Pennsylvania, whose usefulness with the sick was continually sought, I early conceived a liking for, and sought every opportunity to be in a position to relieve the sufferings of others. Later in life I devoted my time, when best I could, to nursing as a business, serving under different doctors for a period of eight years (from '52 to '60); most of the time at my adopted home in Charlestown, Middlesex County, Massachusetts. From these doctors I received letters commending me to the faculty of the New England Female Medical College, whence, four years afterward, I received the degree of Doctress of Medicine. I then practised in Boston, but desiring a larger scope for general information, I travelled toward the British Dominion. On my return, after the close of the Confederate War, my mind centred upon Richmond, the capital city of Virginia, as the proper field for real missionary work, and one that would present ample opportunities to become acquainted with the diseases of women and children.

During my stay there nearly every hour was improved in that sphere of labor. The last quarter of the year 1866, I was enabled, through the agency of the Bureau under Gen. Brown, to have access each day to a very large number of the indigent, and others of different classes, in a population of over 30,000 colored. At the close of my services in that city I returned to my former home, Boston, where I entered into the work with renewed vigor, practising outside, and receiving children in the house for treatment; regardless, in a measure, of remuneration. Although not now in a locality where my constant attendance is required, I do not fail to notice the various published records of the condition of the health of Boston and vicinity.

That woman should study the mechanism of the human structure to better enable her to protect life, before assuming the office of nurse, few will agree. But that good service has been performed by those who were entirely ignorant of it, every one must admit. In my own experience, there was much that to me was obscure, yet, strange to say, I never met with an accident, A kind Father directed every thought in behalf of the helpless.

I believe matrimony to be a divine institution; and that the results arising from a union of the sexes should be considered an important study for each party concerned. If we as intelligent beings sit still in this matter of physical security, premature decay must take the place of perfection. Since I have, with no small degree of diffidence, consented to submit my long-kept journal to the public in the form of a book, I desire to present the different subjects by the use of as few technical terms as possible; and to make my statements brief, simple, and comprehensive. Indeed I desire that my book shall be as a primary reader in the hands of every woman; and yet none the less suited to any who may be conversant with all branches of medical science. If women are permitted to read and reflect for themselves, it is hardly possible that they will say it is uninteresting to them, or that it should only be read by men.

In dealing with subjects that bring to mind thousands of premature mortalities, as, for instance, those from cholera infantum or pneumonia, I deem it expedient to speak only of what I know and to which I can testify. I have endeavored to give some domestic or ready palliative reliefs for the several cases described; thereby hoping to avoid the possibility of a remedy's being applied without an acquaintance with the character and phases of the complaint for which it is intended. There is no doubt that thousands of little ones annually die at our very doors, from diseases which could have been prevented, or cut short by timely aid. People do not wish to feel that death ensues through neglect on their part; indeed they speak of consumption, cholera infantum, and diphtheria, etc., as if sent by God to destroy our infants.

They seem to forget that there is a *cause* for every ailment, and that it may be in their power to remove it. My chief desire in presenting this book is to impress upon somebody's mind the possibilities of prevention.

PART FIRST:

Creating of the cause,
prevention, and cure of infantile
bowel complaints,
from birth to the close
of the teething period,
or till after the fifth year

CHAPTER I.

HOW TO MARRY

AT WHAT AGE should a girl marry? is a question frequently asked by young girls of some confiding friend, and almost as frequently unsatisfactorily answered. Suppose the question be amended thus: – At what age and *how* should young girls marry? The answer to the last clause I would say, taking all things into consideration, with the consent of parents or guardians, it is best for a young woman to accept a suitor who is respectable, vigorous, industrious, and but a few years her senior, if not of an equal age. One who gives evidence, previous to wedlock, of being both capable and willing to take the entire responsibility of a wife upon himself. No objections, of course, to a union with wealth, all other things being equal. No sickly, sensitive young girl need expect to have it all sunshine, even with an industrious, wellmeaning man for a husband, rich or poor. The age of a young woman should be about 19 or 20. It should be remembered that the union of persons of premature growth, that is before the body is well developed on either side, favors weakly children. And the same is true of the union of persons far advanced in years. Weakly mixtures also produce delicate children. A union of persons whose parents are of unmixed blood, and whose statures are nearly in proportion, usually turns out well. A man's age should be between 22 and 25 when taking the responsibility of a family upon him. I will add just here that the way to be happy after marriage is to continue in the careful routine of the courting days, till it becomes a well understood thing between the two.

After marriage, if medical aid is required by the wife, let it be sought in a direction that there will never be cause to regret. Some women are over anxious for a family, and by their nervous whims make themselves and those around them unhappy. But it is to be deplored that there is a much larger class of young women whose minds are dark on the subject of preservation of health, and who soon forget, if they ever thought of the liabilities of a married life. On taking cold or feeling languid or nauseated a physician must at once be sent for. It should be borne in mind that many women begin to show signs of pregnancy by cold, severe pain in the head, back, stomach, or various parts of the body.

Numbers begin and continue for months with severe cramp colic, and if remedies of a powerful nature are applied, the mischief may be alarming. Many of the teas, sweats, baths, and potions that are effective in relieving a cold will be wholly ineffective when pregnancy is certain. Therefore repeated trials but disturbs the nervous system of the mother, through which all things are transmitted to the living germ. In all cases of suppression of the monthly flow after marriage, a careful physician should be at once consulted, if there is any reason to doubt that it is caused by pregnancy. Suffice it to say that too frequent physicking and over-indulgence in intoxicating liquors and tobacco, will cause sickly diminutive offspring, to say nothing of" premature births.

CHAPTER II.

THE PRESENT MODES OF WASHING AND DRESSING THE NEW-BORN

USUALLY, as soon as the birth of a child is an-nounced, a basin or tub of hot water is ordered. The washing begins with a "wee bit of rag" and a great cake of perfumed soap purchased long, long before, for the occasion. Then follows wiping with a great linen towel, during which time the creature gets well aired, being indirectly exhibited to as many as have courage to look on and admire "the cunning little thing."

"The water must be hot, to get off the grease," said an old nurse. Aye, but with ignorant help would it be surprising if a little of the skin came off first? In more favored circles a nice bath tub is prepared, the water of an equal temperature with the room. Some fine soap is put in to make a suds, which is applied after the surface of the body is oiled. Some cold water adherents persist in using ice-cold water upon a new-born babe, depending on "rubbing it to get up a circulation." I once knew a divine (divines have rules sometimes) whose customs led him to have his only child washed in this way, and believing in the adage of "the hair of the dog curing the bite," he continued to doctor it himself for eighteen months, from its birth to its death, with cold water. The babe received a severe cold, stopping up its nostrils and air tubes, and rendering its little life wholly miserable. To the cause of all this suffering they gave the technical name, Catarrh.

The methods of washing infants just described are more common even in this enlightened age of humanity than is generally known. The excuse for cold baths may exist in the mode of life of the erratic tribes, or among uncivilized nations whose minds are dark upon the construction and office of a nervous system. The several sad results that I myself have witnessed at times, and places, that it was not deemed my business to speak, have led me to adopt what seemed a more humane course. With the use of cold water some judgment is required, as many infants, when born, are weak, and ready to yield up life upon the application of the slightest sedative. The skin being so largely supplied with nerves which transmit all sensations to the internal organs, as telegraph wires do the electric current. Thus cold water may send a chill to some vital part, the result of which no effort in the power of man can counteract. It is next to impossible to keep a babe as warm as it should be going through with the customary routine. Indeed it is not at all uncommon for a babe to be laid beside its mother (if not alone in a crib) lips purple and cold as a lump of clay. I once looked upon a babe who from this cause had for three days resisted all attempts to get it warm. Thus, I fear, many come and go. Does any desire to preserve the vitality of a new being? Then it will not suffice to be too self-assured or too oriental to seek to improve in the matter.

I deeply regret to have to state that I have heard many apparently intelligent persons express opposition to the continuation of the human species. But let me ask. What devastating visitations may we not expect if we seek to diminish God's images by any selfish or misguided motives?

THE USE OF SOAP

There are many kinds of soap in use for the purpose of washing clothes, cleansing paint, etc. Then there are not a few advertised as superior for washing the skin. But the fact that water into which soap is rubbed turns white, or becomes sudsy, is sufficient evidence that it contains an alkali, or something having the nature of potash. To use it on the tender skin of infants is but to experiment for the benefit of the dealer, at the expense of the babe. Again, soap is irritating to the more tender surfaces, as the lips and eyelids. If the suds is sucked by the child while the sponge is passed over the face, severe purging may occur. Then if soap gets in the eyes, it is liable to cause sore or inflamed eyes, perhaps for life. I truly believe that more children are afflicted with sore eyes, ears, noses, and heads, whose friends took the precaution to have them washed with "pure baby soap," than could be counted in a hundred years. The germs of bronchitis, which means cold settled in the air-tubes leading to the lungs, – pneumonia, which means lung fever, indigestion, each or all, can be inducted into the system in the first washing. The male physician, unlike the woman physician, does not always remain long enough to see this important duty properly performed. This may be owing to the fact that, among the poorer classes, two or three women are present who are expected to be experts in baby-washing. But, as a fact, many old women sit around on such occasions who have almost as little knowledge what and how to do, as the babe whose expected advent has called them together. Therefore we cannot too strongly protest against the practice of many physicians, – that of leaving a woman in the hands of an inexperienced person as soon as the navel cord is severed. For it is not at all reasonable to conclude, that because a woman is the mother of many children, she is an expert in the matter of washing and dressing the newborn, or of relieving the various ailments incident upon child-bearing.

CHAPTER III.

PREPARATIONS FOR CONFINEMENT

WHEN A WOMAN is expected to be sick, if a physician has not been engaged as one should have been, no time should be lost in seeking quietly to notify one. It is just as important that a doctor should be in attendance before the birth of a poor woman's child as that he should be present before the birth of the child of wealth. And it should be considered inhuman in any physician to purposely absent him or herself until after the birth of the child. With a little benevolence and perseverance, the most humble in life can be provided with bedstead and bedding, upon which should be fixed securely pads of cotton batting, or woollen cloths. Also there should be provided clean apparel for a change of under-garments, should such change be needful. The chemise and gown should be well taken up so as to be kept dry; as wet or soiled bedding or apparel in time of labor is a frequent cause of severe chills. For the same reason, should instruments or vessels be warmed before inserting, in the case of instrumental labors. The surrounding atmosphere should be comfortable, never too warm or too cold. When there is no physician present, and a child is so fortunate as to "born itself," surely some one can be found to assist it to survive the task. After cautiously looking under cover to see that the infant's face is clear from contact of any parts or particles, patience will aid in determining how best to complete a well-begun job.

BORN WITH A CAUL

It is no uncommon thing, in hasty labor, for the bag of water to break and remain close around the face and neck of the child. This is done by the quick, rolling motion in coming into the world. The force of the descent breaks the thin skin or bag, and the same force packs the face into it; so that it remains over the face, partly around the neck, and sometimes over the head as well Were it not removed, the child must suffocate. This circumstance at a birth has given rise to the sayings, "Born with a caul," "Born with a veil," etc. The proper way to remove this bag or membrane is, from over the head down, as lifting it may pull open the eyes; thereby bringing the eyeball in contact with the fluid or the chalk-like substance, thus laying the foundation for sore eyes. After twenty minutes or more, beating having ceased in the cord, – which may be known by pressing closely between the fingers that part nearest the belly of the child, – it should be tied by means of a flat knot, with lamp wicking, or many strands of white spool cotton, about a finger's length from the belly. In case of twins, there should be a second tie the same length from the first, and the cord cut between the two ties. There have been times when women depended largely upon each other, in their helpless hours of confinement; it may be so again, but with a far greater chance of successful results.

———

CHAPTER IV.

THE BETTER MODE OF WASHING THE NEW-BORN

WASHING IS the name given to the old method. Cleansing is the proper one for the new.

How to proceed: A soft, white, all wool blanket, about two yards square, should be always in readiness when a birth is expected. Not necessarily new, but pure, never having been used about fever patients, or about the dead. A metallic slop-pail with cover, that all secundine particles may be put out of sight; the same serving as a vessel for the woman to sit over. As soon as the babe is freed from the mother, it should be wrapped in the blanket and laid aside in a comfortable place. After the mother's safety is assured of, prepare thus to clean and dress the babe: Secure a comfortable position, with plenty of light and ventilation, as far from the confinement bed as possible. Have a stand or covered chair, upon which to place the half of a small teacupful of fresh hog's lard or sweet oil. If in a cold room, warm the grease by setting the cup in hot water for a few minutes. Have a piece of soft, all-wool flannel, about the size of your pocket-handkerchief, another piece half as large, and two pieces of soft linen or cotton about as large as your hand. A piece of lamp wicking or several strands of white spool cotton, to be used in re-tying, in case of bleeding from the cut end of the cord. The infant may then be brought forth, held on the lap, or laid on two chairs. As many babes have open eyes as soon born, it is best to dip a small piece of the soft linen or cotton in the grease, and wipe the inner edges of the lids first of all, as the drying on of the chalky substance or other matter with which the child's face may have had contact, while coming into the world, may, as I have before said, be the first cause of sore or inflamed eyes. Then proceed with the small piece of flannel, well saturated with oil, to clean the face, ears, nose, – avoiding the eyes, – neck, chest, under the arms and between the fingers. Wipe dry with the clean, large piece of flannel. Those parts can then be covered with a part of the blanket, and the lower extremities cleaned with care. Should there be dried Wood from the cut end of the cord, moisten with warm water, and wipe it off. Then proceed to clean and examine well all the private parts. When done, cut a hole in the piece of cotton, linen or batting, as it may suit, about the size of your hand, through which slip the cord, fold it closely, but flat and smooth, and lay it over to the left side of the belly, that it may not intercept the circulation of the liver, which is situated on the right side. Then secure it with an all-wool flannel band. The band should be made so as to include a shirt with long sleeves. It should extend from over the teats down below the hips. There never would be swelling of the breasts of infants if the bands were purposely made wide. The natural office of the mama in girl-children, has been destroyed by repeated pressing of the teats with the mistaken purpose of "getting out the milk." Narrow bands are worthless. If they shrink they should be pieced out or replaced with new. The band securely placed, – a flannel roller, plain slip and napkin, is all that is required for the first dressing. It often happens that, after "washing" and dressing by present methods, blood oozes from the cut end of the cord. Seldom docs this happen by the new method, – I should say, my method. Sometimes the fault is in the manner of tying, or from imperfection of the cord itself. In any case the cord should be re-tied, or the bleeding otherwise stopped, and the infant kept warm till medical aid can be summoned. To return to first dressing: After the wraps have been drawn up over the feet, the head should be thoroughly greased and cleaned, taking care not to press the bones in the least. Pressure upon the head at birth may be the means of stupidity, or even idiocy, during life. The baby's mouth should then be swabbed out with a clean, wet cloth, and the little one laid down in quiet. Babies usually sleep during the procedure, as does the mother, she waking only to find her babe by her side, "all warm, sweet and clean," and " mamma didn't even hear it cry once." One trial of this method is convincing of its benefits. If soap is used with grease, it acts the same as suds into which new cotton cloth is put. No good laundress will meet with such an accident, if possible to avoid it. And surely no careful nurse will allow her little charge to suffer by having to stop and change the water. Moreover, in the absence of soap, there is no liability to chapped skin, glandular sores, sore eyes, ears, and crusty scalp. Especially should the scalp be well cleaned, and kept so; as it not only adds to the tidy appearance of the child, but favors an even, healthy growth of the hair bulbs. The foundation for a love of cleanliness can best be laid in infancy. There are many adults who desire good hair, yet do not or will not know that combing the hair daily, and keeping the scalp clean and cool, promotes a healthy growth of the hair.

———

CHAPTER V.

NECESSITY OF AGREEABLE
AND SOOTHING SURROUNDINGS

NO BAY RUM, perfume, puff powders or other unnatural substances should be tolerated about young infants, But after the patients have been made comfortable, all soiled clothing or slops should be quietly removed. All loud talking or laughing should be strictly prohibited. To insure this, no sly jokes should be indulged in by any one present; for by so doing convulsions of an alarming nature may be brought on. Judging from the actions of some women, when around a confinement bed, it is not at all unlikely that many cases of internal convulsions, both of mother and child, are the results of inward or suppressed laughter soon after delivery, and before the womb has had time to get in place, or when the babe is nursing.

Infants should be accustomed to a change of apparel as soon as possible. It is an error to suppose that a child should be kept hot, and tucked down in soiled wrappings till after the navel drops off. After twenty-four hours it can be wiped with clean warm water, close around the navel.

The napkins, too, should be changed and washed out just as often as soiled. Also there should be clean day wraps and night slips in constant readiness during the child's helpless period. Heavy or wadded coverlets should be discarded, even in the coldest weather, for the reason that they are heavier than woollen, retain the moisture from breaths, are not so easily washed as woollen blankets, nor are they so warm. The science of our nature teaches us that woollen is the best covering during the hours of sleep. For instance, the pores of our skin permit the escape of all gases not necessary for the renewal of the tissues of the body; in like manner woollen goods permit the odors to escape from our bodies.

The face of an infant should never be covered when asleep, especially when in the bed with adults; it induces lung difficulties. The blood must pass through the heart and lungs, uninterrupted, day and night, in order to supply all parts of the body. The hours for sleep are intended for the repair of worn material, while at the same time the useless matter is passing off in breath or perspiration. I believe that all infants should be supplied with a light covering for the head day and night, until the hair grows out. The old style lace cap, for instance, deserves a conspicuous place among the relics of health preservers. Later on, the hair becomes the only proper covering for the head day or night. By all means, a child should be closely watched, and its wraps changed and adapted to atmospherical changes. If infants are too tightly wrapped, or are allowed to get too hot, they generally make it known by writhing or whining in their sleep.

By using oil in the first cleaning the temperature of the child's body is not much changed. I do not propose to describe any of the abnormal liabilities of the cord circulation, that might require the use of hot or cold water, in order to save life. As medical advice should be sought in all doubtful or unnatural cases, the unnatural can only be known by close attention to the appearance of the natural.

———

CHAPTER VI.

NURSING FROM THE BREAST MADE EASY

AFTER the lapse of two or three hours, the mother is likely to feel concerned for her child; but, should both incline to be quiet, neither should be awakened for the purpose of nursing. Too early an attempt to put the child to the breast is frequently the cause of much unnecessary pain to the mother. Before a child is put to the breast, all soiled linen must be removed from the mother, the face, neck, breasts, hands, and under the arms well wiped with a cloth wrung out of warm water, then covered with a clean flannel chemise open at the nipple. Bay Rum may be added to the water if required. The private parts should be well wiped under cover, greased with lard, and covered with a large, warm napkin, after which a wide bandage should be buttoned on. The babe will not suffer by waiting. The greater number of women afford milk enough in a few hours to supply the needs of their young. The exceptions being either from some malformation or a watery condition of the blood. When the milk pores are free, the child can obtain enough to satisfy it in a short time. If, on the contrary, the glands are hard or unbroken, as they most always are in case of a first child, it becomes the indispensable duty of the nurse to soften the glands, and start the milk running; as it is impossible for the babe to do it by a few draws with its tongue. The glands may be softened by the following means: Besmear the hands with warm goose or olive oil, and anoint the breasts slowly and evenly from under the arms down to the nipple, until the glands soften and the milk begins to flow; after which nipple cups should be kept on in the intervals of nursing. Chapped or bleeding nipples may be cured by frequent sponging off with warm salt water. If through neglect an abscess gets ahead, it should be encouraged to suppurate in one spot, by the application of warm poultices of flaxseed meal, salt, hops, or honey and flour, and when ripe opened with the lancet; the babe continuing to suck through the artificial teat.

Those manufactured by Robert R. Kent are invaluable.

If, after the milk has appeared, the glands harden and the milk veins become knotty and painful, I also make use of the following means to relieve quickly: Steep half an ounce of Indian Posy, or Life Everlasting herb, in a pint of water. Oil the hands, and bathe in the same way I have described, with the decoction as hot as can be borne, the patient being in an easy, half sitting posture. In the intervals of rest, she should drink a teacupful quite hot, with or without sugar. When the tumor is considerably advanced, the process of breaking it up is often very painful, and may even cause fainting; but relief is sure if the work is patiently performed and courageously endured. The pain of that is light compared to the torture, for weeks together, of abscesses. The herb has no more specific action than that of relaxing the system through the aid of the absorbents or sweat glands. It relaxes the skin, and is safe to drink as a diet to increase the flow of milk. A child may be born perfectly healthy, yet even for days be slow to take hold of the nipple; whereas many seize hold at once. The friends fret and declare the babe is starving, if it does not desire to suck. If they could only read the meaning in those little eyes as they open and shut, they would know the secret – rest, simply rest, preparatory to the task. Many young mothers have no prominence to the nipple, so that neglect on the part of the nurse may cause such to lose the benefits of suckling. A friendly adult or child could soon draw out the nipple by sucking so that the babe can get hold; after which the nipple cups should be kept in constant use, till the babe is strong enough to keep the glands soft, and the nipple pliable. Usually, at this juncture, all sorts of teas are suggested: molasses water, milk and sugar and water; and should the child dare to cry, after the plentiful administration of one or all these teas, up steps an experienced old friend, or grandma, who declares that it must have "catnip tea." So the world-renowned catnip tea is authoritatively given, while are related the many cases in which the drug was known to have cured wind colic, and how it quiets and fattens generally. Only when the child belches, and refuses to let any more go down its throat, does the pouring in cease. And even this is sometimes taken as an indication that the babe is full, and needs to be trotted to make room for more. Some babes are eager to suck at .birth, even seizing hold of the sponge as it passes the mouth in washing the face. If babes are not fed just when they fret and whine, some knowing ones say they "suck wind." Well, is it not natural that they should suck wind, since they are in the world If they are allowed to lie quietly for a few hours, and are then given a few drops of sweet cream or milk, without sugar, they will give scarcely any trouble, and in due time nature will furnish strength to obtain with ease the amount of nourishment suitable to the delicate organs of digestion. It frequently happens that a babe has a rattling or wheezing noise in its throat, or air tubes; in such cases, a feather has usually been recommended with which to tickle the back part of the tongue. I always wet the feather, to lay the down. The tickling excites a coughing or gagging, which dislodges the phlegm, so that it can be hooked out with the finger. There are reasons for suspecting that many new-born infants have strangled to death from this cause. I do not mean to cast any reflections when I say that a physician is not likely to be informed of the fact, until it is too late to remove the difficulty. And as the wheezing may assume the same sound as that of catarrh, cold in the air-tubes, bronchitis or croup, the real cause may be lost sight of. Promptness is all that is required when any such trouble presents. The fumes of tobacco, whiskey, smoking lamps or stoves, – also wetting the nipple with spittle when eating snuff, each of these may not only be disagreeable to a young infant, but may sicken it and cause instant death. It is true, however, that many children have survived all of these disadvantages, but who can tell how much has been taken from their health, and length of days. Infants should be nursed frequently at first, to give them a good start; they seldom suck more than they need. But from the beginning they should be fed, then laid down. As they grow older they will nurse well, and expect to lie down afterwards. Early and regular habits of nursing prevent the liability to mammary abscesses, ovarian or uterine tumors. Hence, suckling a child as soon as convenient after birth, not only serves to quicken the vitality of the new being by cleansing the bowels and supplying new blood, but it also serves to clear out the system of the mother.

CHAPTER VII.

THE USELESSNESS OF "BABY MEDICINES" DURING THE MONTH

PROBABLY the greatest amount of mischief arising from the administration of " baby teas," lies in the fact that they are not given with the least certainty as to their effect upon the system of the child, whether to nourish the blood or physic the bowels. Let us take catnip: this' is a herb described in some books as being a mild laxative, good to work off cold on the chest and bowels of infants; a sweat-promoter. About a dozen years ago a neighbor of one of my patients, thinking it for the best, gave catnip tea to her three-days'-old son. I was hastily summoned, and on arriving in the room where everything a few hours before was so tranquil, I suspected that catnip tea had been around. Of course no one would own up until, after I had staid by the little victim fifteen hours without sleep, finally succeeding in checking the frequent green discharges and thus saving the child's life, – shame, caused the disclosure of the cause of the mischief. The tea had not been given for food, as the mother had a full supply; but as the babe was moving about, it was thought that a little catnip tea would make it sleep. A lady told me with great dignity that her children ate homoeopathic pills when they wished. "Why," said she, " my children fatten on them."

I saw that she did not know the secret of the "fattening." Another said, "Why, my James eats castor-oil on bread." Now we are aware that there are very many articles used as food that can be prepared and combined so as to act in place of medicine in certain cases; but as a general thing medicine will not answer to nourish the body in place of food. According to the mechanism of man, there are three stages in his life for which due preparation is made, before he comes into existence, to wit: the breasts' milk for infancy, the teeth, with which to eat solid food, and medicine, to heal when sick. As to catnip producing sleep, I cannot agree with old ladies in general; but I do know of a truth that if a child is dosed with it in early infancy, the effect is to loosen the bowels; the fatigue from this over-distension of the stomach causes sleep. Babes should move about if they have life enough in them; they should, by no means, be stupefied. The first milk from the breast is the only medicine needed; when other mixtures are poured into the child's stomach, as teas sweetened with sugar, honey, molasses, either of which is laxative, the danger is greatly augmented, especially if given before the bowels have moved at all. The custom of old-fashioned people, as they style themselves, of giving new-born babes castor-oil and molasses, or soot tea (for that irrepressible belly-ache), and urine and molasses, to clean them out, is, though with reluctance, fast dying out. It would be well to notice that children who are dosed during infancy for every supposed ill are seldom robust. They become physically stunted, and their peevish habits exact for them all sorts of over-indulgence. More food for the blood, and less medicine, should be the motto. Let us follow the tide of progression. There are no uniform rules by which infants are to have a discharge at birth, either from the bowels or bladder. Therefore, no efforts to induce such should be used until necessity demands it. It is no uncommon thing for infants to pass large quantities from the bowels, just as they are entering the world; a circumstance not likely to be noticed by those unaccustomed to all the incidents of childbirth. It is always safe to await the action of the first food, whether from the breast or artificial; and if it be but a few drops well digested, there need be no fear but that the napkins will be soiled as fast as desired. If such result does not follow, after waiting two or three days, a flannel cloth folded, and wrung out of hot water, laid first on your cheek, then on the child's belly, and that covered with dry flannel, will, with perseverance, bring about the desired result. Sometimes an infant passes large quantities of the dark matter immediately after the fatigue of washing and dressing (old style); then it may pass no more for two or three days, or until time has been given for matter to accumulate. If the organs of the child are all right, all will be well. But should doubts arise as to the best course to take, surely medical advice only needs the seeking. It was formerly the custom, and is now to a great extent with old nurses, to give later in the month – certainly before their month was up, as all teas and charms had to be given before they left – saffron tea. I have seen them sit by a hot stove and feed infants with saffron tea more patiently than they would like it given to them. I once asked a high-priced nurse why she gave saffron tea. I was kindly, though decidedly, informed that it was to "push the gums." I was none the wiser by asking. I afterward learned from the child's older sister that the doctor said the baby had the jaundice. Weir it might have the jaundice, kept in a room with a temperature of 80 degrees, with two adult persons night and day, and fed on saffron tea. Now the crocus, or saffron, sometimes grown in our gardens, is described as possessing sweating properties, being good to promote eruptions of the skin in fevers, and good in fits. Yet thousands of infants, no doubt, have been forced to swallow saffron tea, who have not given the slightest evidence of any unnatural complaint. No paregoric, laudanum, or other preparations containing opium, should ever be given to an infant for the purpose of quieting or making it sleep. Sleep-producers serve only to bind the bowels and stupefy the senses. Carminatives – medicines that expel wind – such as caraway, fennel, anise, cardamon, mints and the like, should never be given unless prescribed by those competent to vouch for their effect.

It is becoming a widespread custom to send a little girl or boy to a druggist's to purchase some advertised baby medicine or food. The patent cough syrups, or those kept on hand in shops, I deem unsafe in the hands of the inexperienced. Most, if not all of them, contain some sleepproducing ingredient, whereby they may check a cough by paralyzing, as it were, the little nerves of sensation in the air tubes; thus giving opportunity for the phlegm to collect in great quantities, with no possible way of escape. Doubtless in this way suffocation is frequently induced, in whoopingcough, bronchitis, or croup.

Several years ago, in the city of Boston, a mother returned from work, and found her baby, which she had left alone, a corpse. Her explanation, as it appeared in the daily papers, was to the effect that she had given the child the rinsings of the vial that contained laudanum, to keep it quiet.

People are getting much wiser nowadays; laudanum and paregoric cannot be easily obtained without a recipe. But they can yet buy and give large doses of "Patent Soothing Syrups."

In all cases of difficult breathing or signs of croup, with or without hot skin, a soft flannel cloth should be wrung out of hot water, and laid over the entire chest, close up under the chin and ears; and if the bowels are bound, it may extend to the belly, the whole being covered with a dry, warm flannel. By this means the force of a cold can be broken, the breathing relieved, and in a majority of cases it is all that is required to be done. Even in severe cases of lung fever, warm water applications are invaluable; acting as an absorbent through the medium of the pores of the skin. If a paste of flax-seed meal is used, it should be applied in the same way. If the applications are to be warm, they should be kept warm, and if they are to be cold, should be kept cold, until relief is obtained.

I may have digressed somewhat, as pneumonia seldom develops in the first month of infancy. At all events, external applications are in place till medical aid is secured. I do not wish to be understood as usurping the power of other physicians; each has his or her own method of procedure.

I merely wish to impress the domestic and common sense means, to be used in cases of emergency.

The old custom of giving infants " a little weak toddy" to "bring up the wind and make them sleep," should henceforth and forever be removed from the midst of a more enlightened people. If it is given weak the effect is to intoxicate at first, and then produce sleep; which may be followed by a fearful attack of purging. If given strong, it may induce constipation and dry colic, the very thing it is intended to relieve. Such a course may also have inculcated a desire for tippling in many of our weak-minded youth. Castor-oil is a wellknown sickening purgative, and it does seem to be a wonderful interposition of Providence alone, that so many thousand infants have survived the compulsory dosing with this drug. But a few years ago a lady, aged about sixty-five, came to her end from severe diarrhea, brought on, as she testified, by taking a "store-bottle of castor-oil at a dose."

Mothers and nurses should strive to become familiar with all articles of diet; also with the properties and medical uses of all drugs and minerals, and their action upon the animal economy.

———————

CHAPTER VIII.

DROPPING OF THE NAVEL CORD

IT WOULD more than pay me, if in this section I could say aught that would effect the removal of the anxiety generally shown concerning the healing of the navel.

There is a late custom recommended by some physician, that of soaking of the lint, to apply clean each day. This, in my judgment, is risking too much, unless it be with the guidance of an experienced person. I deem it much safer to wipe close around the wound daily; then on the third day slip a clean piece of soft cotton or linen beneath and around the soiled pad; as about this time the cord, unless very thick, is dry and will soon drop off, leaving the clean pad as a protecting ring around the navel. The navel should then be looked after each day until healed. But it is an error to suppose that the navel should be healed in any certain number of days. The usual time is from five to seven days; but I have known many to drop on the third day, and more to remain unhealed till after the twelfth or fourteenth day. In the former case the cords were very small; in the latter they were very large and strong.

Many years ago, I learned of an accident that occurred to a midwife of much usefulness: Because the cord remained eight days, she cut what she supposed was a piece of thread; in consequence of which the child bled to death. It would be well to state here that keeping the babe too hot retards the drying of the umbilical vessels. Ordinarily the healing of the navel is simple and natural, and it should never be tampered with. Should unnatural growths appear, any regular physician can detect the cause, and direct the cure at once. Far more accidents occur by the reluctance of friends around to call medical aid in time, than from the cause itself. Selfish prudence is too often allowed to come between duty and human life. If at any time a white fluid should be discharged from the vagina, or private parts, of a girl child, it should be washed away as often as seen, and the parts washed out with a solution of common salt I have seen mothers become greatly frightened at this common occurrence. Cleanliness and perseverance will remove the trouble. If families would make it a rule to have a thermometer in the nursery or the sleeping-room, by which to regulate the temperature of the body, many of these baby-ills would be banished from our midst. The nervous system of babes deserves a large share of our sympathy. But if one were to judge from the treatment they sometimes undergo, it might be inferred that, like dolls, infants have no nerves or rights which men are bound to respect. Children of the same family differ much. One may be sprightly, making frequent music by crying; the other may be comparatively docile. And if a child is quiet and does not cry, or act silly, it is called stupid, and everything is done to arouse its ire.

Children cry for pastime; so they should. It develops the lungs and relieves the air-tubes of any collections of phlegm. Besides, it causes them to be noticed by some one who might forget their existence. There cannot be any comfort in being rocked, tossed, shook and kissed, and that, too, without any regard to the odor of the breath. It is decidedly injurious to wake babes from a quiet sleep, or even to excite their attention while lying quiet. Mothers should early learn to listen and become familiar with the different tones produced in the cries even of the same child. Listening should be cultivated more; then the possibility of making a crying baby more noisy, by shocking it with additional noises, will need no more explanation. " Oh," says one, " they get used to it and look for it." True, – bred, born, aye and raised in excitement; never can hear or understand anything but noise, noise, noise.

Currents of cold air from a window or door should not be permitted to pass over the exposed body of infants; as, by so doing, the sudden change may, like electricity, direct the irritation to some vital organ. It is considered much safer, when the weather permits, to put on suitable wraps and take them in the open air. The most trouble arises from keeping the infant too warm from birth. Hot-house plants rarely endure the changes of the open air, until it becomes equal to what they have been used to.

———

CHAPTER IX.

ARTIFICIAL NURSING

SHOULD the mother afford no milk by reason of malformation, or otherwise, the child should be accustomed to the most healthful kind of food from the first. Milk from one animal should be sought. Animals that are fed on corn, hay and fodder, make the best milk in winter; those fed on clover and cured hay, the best in summer. The milk of animals fed mostly on turnips, cabbages, and potatoes, is more apt to disagree with the stomach.

The goat furnishes an even diet for infants, but its milk is not so easy to obtain in large cities.

Milk should be given to a child in its purity, not deprived of the cream or watered. Watering is equal to skimming, and vice versa. And when the child has never known the taste of its mother's milk, I can see no philosophy in directing the milk to be watered and sweetened to make it taste like breast-milk.

All attempts to increase the quantity of babes' food by watering are indeed robbery, as relates to the infants; such weakening should only be practised for special reasons. But to insure success, pure milk, or cream with some water, should be the rule, not the exception.

In a warm atmosphere the milk or cream should be made scalding hot by setting it in a vessel of boiling water, and stirring it the while. Boiling deprives it of the cream and other nutritive properties. There should be no more warmed than is to be used up. The warming should be by putting the milk in the bottle, then placing the latter in hot water a few minutes. In this way the quality and temperature of the drink remains uniform. The capacity of the bottle selected should be about one ounce. The material of which the black elastic nipple is composed, is not supposed to injure the mouth. No sugar should be added.

Babes have been raised to a fine size on various kinds of porridge; and they can be supported by putting a piece of clean linen into the shape of a teat, fastening a soft string about it so that it may be held by the nurse or any one, while food is poured into it from a spoon. Many are the times that I have fed them in that way. I never thought of laying them down to feed themselves.

Milk may be used just as it comes from the animal; it is only in cases where it is kept on hand for a day that it really need be scalded.

So much emphasis has been put upon the necessity of water as a constituent of baby diet, that it is almost venturing too far to remind any of the fact that most milk dealers are careful that this constituent shall be already supplied.

Formerly, dropsical, emaciated, half-starved, fretful babes were very numerous; but since, of late, judicious legislation has been brought to bear on the matter of adulterating milk, things have changed.

Henceforth we may hope to hear that infantile deaths from this probable cause decrease annually.

With meagre feeding a "bouncing fat boy" will soon present the appearance of a wrinkled old man. And, too, the condition in which food is presented to a child is equally as important as the quality and quantity. It is impossible to rule the stomach of another; a spunky child will resent the attempt some way, and at some time, even though it be after the injury is irreparable. A uniformity in heating the milk or food of any kind is very important. Hot things should never enter a babe's mouth. If milk is in the least sour, it is running a great risk to try to sweeten it by adding soda, as some persons do, for convenience.

The coarse habit of "stuffing" babes, to avoid frequent feeding of them, should vanish like dew before the noonday sun; us it probably will, under the management of educated mothers and nurses. The old-fashioned way of compelling babes to suck a "sugar teat" or a piece of fat meat rind for hours together to keep them quiet, is cheating, to say the least. Our domestic fowls will eat meal, grain and vegetables when they can get them. And if all supply of food is cut off, they may be seen to pick, pick, day after day; this they will do if the ground is frozen and bare. But are they getting food? Nay, they are only tasting, smelling, and hunting for food.

Sucking a sugar teat or meat rind, like gumchewing, tends to undermine the natural vigor of the mind, by a waste of the fluids that are intended to prepare the food for making pure blood.

A child can just as kindly be fed, changed, and laid quietly to rest; it does not need patting or rocking.

Baby-raising is made irksome by adults themselves. The feeding and putting to sleep should be superintended by some competent person, as by intrusting it to children, or even young girls, the feeding may be imperfect. Many children scream with fright at the noise created to get them to sleep.

Canned or otherwise prepared baby -food is quite uncertain, unless, in the case of canned milk, particular pains is taken to have the water hot, and the mass well dissolved; a large part will remain at the bottom of the vessel. Again, as there is more than one brand of this article, it is hard to find out which is the purest, as all are advertised to be the best. Of course the largest firm will have the largest sales. Then the price is not so convenient at all times, rather encouraging the habit of rinsing the can; while all infants' food should be prepared fresh when wanted.

Some babes spit up their food from the first, but there is nothing alarming about that. Should what is spit up smell sour, and appear indigested, small doses of pulverized magnesia – say about as much as will lay on a five-cent silver piece – will correct it, while any known cause should be removed at once. In case of purging in early infancy, it is a mistake not to stop it as soon as possible. It is always safe, after removing the cause, to quiet the motion of the bowels; a thing which can be done only by proper scientific means, that no one should fail to secure.

———

CHAPTER X.

THE MILK FEVER

VERY many women have milk in the breasts before the birth of a child. Others do not have any for some days after confinement, yet may appear comfortable. It is no uncommon thing for them to forget that they have another very important task to perform, – that of preparing healthy meals for the offspring. If, at this time, company is allowed, talking and laughing indulged in, the symptoms of the coming milk may be greatly augmented; so that what might have been a slight chill, headaches or fever may become so severe as to require prompt medical aid. Indeed diarrhea, convulsions, or even insanity may be brought on through the means of any excitement whatever, between the birth of the child and the establishment of the milk.

Giving castor-oil or other nauseous drugs (as has been, and to a great extent is now, the custom) is quite risky, even when prescribed by a physician; as many women are of such a costive habit, that it requires a very large dose to move the bowels. I repeat, it is risking too much, when given in the ordinary ways, for both mother and child. On the part of the mother, an overdose may cause excessive purging and consequent weakness. On the part of the child, should it be nursing while the physicking is going on, the result may be griping and purging, ending its life in a few hours. Every means should be resorted to move the bowels, where such relief is really needful, before administering physic.

Many women have a large passage during the delivery of the child; and therefore need not be disturbed about that matter for days, or even a week, all other things being favorable. For it should be borne in mind that the internal organs are, in a measure, paralyzed by the interruptions of nature during labor, and that time is needed to rest the nerves and bring things in proper order. Headache, so commonly complained of after delivery, is more from exhaustion of the nervous system than from constipation. For this reason should extreme quiet be observed for about nine days. When physic must inevitably be given during the coming of the milk, it is decidedly best to keep the babe from the breast until it is all through with.

But, as a general thing, other means will answer; such as wringing a cloth out of hot water and applying over the abdomen, or belly, rubbing down and across the back and loins, giving large drinks of hot water without sugar, keeping the body warm and moist for a while, but never an injection unless directed by a practitioner.

I would suggest that a few dollars paid to a physician for a half-dozen extra visits during the first weeks of confinement, might prevent months and years of gloom in many families. Again, there are many women that take suddenly ill with vomiting and purging about the time for the milk to appear. The violence with which this trouble progresses, and the depressing consequences by which it is characterized, have indeed caused it to be termed " Child-bed cholera"; and although it may arise from a previously disordered liver or stomach, it seldom happens unless there has been indulgence in suppressed laughing, inhaling peculiar odors, over-eating or drinking. Although the coming of the milk is most commonly ushered in with some degree of chill or fever, there are as many, no doubt, who experience no change whatever, it being so slight. Hence it probably would be best if the term "milk fever" were never used until really apparent. If, after lactation has become perfect, it should go and come, means should be at once resorted to insure its continuance. Wine, ale or beer are not advisable for this purpose. They may surely lead to the habit of moderate intemperance, while their benefits are only temporary. Pure blood is the basis for pure milk, therefore nutritive articles of diet are of more permanent use.

It is well to bear in mind that a scarcity of milk during the month should never be taken as an excuse for refusing to nurse the child; for if it can get but a spoonful a day, it greatly encourages the chance for increasing it. The mother's milk is the fountain of life to the babe, and. therefore seldom dries up unless there be some unnatural obstruction. It has been said by many close observers, that when the milk goes away without some perceptible cause, the child is not to live.

What will cause the milk to disappear in some women, will not in others. Peculiar odors, or pungent, volatile applications will completely and forever drive the milk from the breasts of some women; and a cessation of the milk is frequently a forerunner of consumption of the lungs or tumors about the ovaries. If the nipples crack and bleed, they should be anointed with goose oil, occasionally cold cream, or wet with a solution of sal ammonia, or vinegar and water. This done in the intervals of the babe's sleep, care should be taken to wipe the nipples before offering them to it. When a mother gives up to the thought that the suckling is the hardest part to bear, and impatiently deprives her infant of the breast, the pleasures of life must be to her of small value. "Try, try again," is an adage worth heeding.

Should there be humor in the blood, as there ofttimes is, the nipples will not readily heal while the child nurses; in which case it is advisable to feed the child from a bottle and treat the mother. After relief is obtained, the nursing can be resumed. In ordinary cases a poultice made of bruised burdock root and elm flour, together with a tea made by steeping burdock root and drinking a pint a day; keeping the bowels regular, eating rye and Indian bread, and taking about a half teaspoonful of calcined magnesia dissolved in water, once a day, will effect a cure. The poultice should be made soft and applied fresh twice a day between two thin cloths.

A lady of wealth may get discouraged and give her babe to the care of another, whose babe may in consequence have to be put in some charityhouse or otherwise to board. Her babe may thrive and live; while that of her wet-nurse may soon pine away and die." No one can avoid distressing others unless he strives, to the best of his ability, to bear his own burdens.

CHAPTER XI.

PRECAUTIONS AFTER THE MONTH – PROPER AND IMPROPER DIET

THERE ARE many families in moderate circumstances who, no doubt, feel unable to keep more than one fire going during the cold season; yet nevertheless subject themselves* and children to frequent and severe colds by the sudden change from a hot room to a cold sleeping-apartment. This might in a great measure be prevented by a little extra care to secure tenements with sufficient rooms on one floor.

An infant should never be allowed to take its regular naps in a hot kitchen, amid steam and dust; or in an ironing room, with all of its day-clothes on, beside extra cover, and then be undressed and put to bed in a room that no heat, not even that of the sun, is allowed to enter. Piling on heavy comforters renders the breathing heavy. No baby's face should be covered while asleep. It is wonderful to see how hard some of these little victims struggle to breathe while they sleep, if sleep it can be called.

Some babes kick off the cover, and after being very warm get very cold; to avoid which, soft flannel night-drawers, made so as to include socks and all, should be used.

Comfortable sleeping apartments without fire are healthy. The lungs of grown persons break down from cause of too much pressure, much more infants; yet from all such exciting causes the airtubes may escape, and the liver, stomach or bowels receive the whole mischief.

The sleep of children cannot be healthful if their clothes remain pinned down beneath and around them, and, it may be, tight leather shoes on. Besides, it cultivates untidyness to oblige them to submit to such management. On the contrary, every effort, even at the sacrifice of personal pleasure, should be put forth to insure that clean, sweet and undisturbed repose so much required, and without which few, if any, are perfectly developed.

When it is remembered that from the air we in hale come the principles of life, and how much it is in our power to avoid the contact with injurious particles or substances therein contained, many disadvantages in the matter of rearing the babe will disappear. The air they breathe should be as much one way as possible; no sudden gusts of wind should be forced upon them by hoisting a window when they are over-warm.

Children, of any age, should not be permitted to sleep in the open air, unless it might be for a few minutes, and where the air is extremely bland; which it seldom is, on our New England parks and gardens. A gradual change in the matter of bathing, dressing, feeding, and putting to sleep should be the rule.

The mother may at any time during lactation communicate cold to a child. My first experience in this matter was about thirty-five years ago, when assisting in the care of a child that was nursing. The mother being very warm one summer day, drank freely of ice cold water while the babe of about six months was sucking. She had not much more than time to set the glass down when the babe was seized with rigid convulsions, and dropped from the breast. The mother became almost helpless with fright, and as the next farm was some distance off, I had to use my young brain. Therefore, I procured a tub with some warm water and a little mustard; it may have been a "fearful lot," but the infant was all right when I got through with it.

Over-work or great fatigue in any way should be avoided by women that suckle their children. If obliged to work and scrub, at home or elsewhere, they should endeavor to keep a strict watch over the condition of that life fountain, the breastmilk. There is no known law preventing carefulness.

Again, it is a mistake to indulge in drinking beers or other alcoholic slops to prevent the child's nursing cold. Early subsistence from the strength of whiskey, rum, beers and ales, like tobacco, tends to stunt the intellect and dwarf the stature of the youth of our land. It is much better to eat warm soups, or such solid food as will give permanent warmth to the blood, and insure a clear character to the being. When it is a babe's meal-time, it should be served with the most exquisite care, as upon that depends its proper growth and length of days. To prove this a fact, take, for instance, an old woman or old man upon whom adversity may have made some telling marks in their younger days, and whose days appear nearly at an end, and let such be well cared for in a neat, quiet, comfortable home; the chances are they will live on in brightness of hope for a number of years.

Contrary to the teachings of some so-called missionaries, I believe that neatness in arranging food, dress, or whatever pertains to order and pleasantness, is the most essential part of a Christian duty. For surely if the body is cherished as the image of our Maker, the soul-salvation is a possibility.

I alluded in Chap. II. to putting the new-born in a crib. Not that I oppose their lying alone – on the contrary, I deem it highly conducive both to health and good morals for every one, when at a proper age, to sleep alone.

Now since we have noticed to some extent how sudden emotions, as of grief, anger or fright may shock the child at the breast through the agency of those little organs called nerves, – we will pass on to notice some of the causes of bowel complaints arising from the nature of the food eaten by the nurse. Probably there is no cause more frequently productive of infantile bowel complaints, both during and after the month, than that of the too early indulgence in a mixed diet. It may be well to enumerate some of the more objectionable articles of diet from the first day of confinement to the seventh or ninth month, or time for weaning. Of the vegetables, – beans, dry or green, cabbage, cooked or raw, beets, turnips, cucumbers, green peas, dandelions, spinach and Carolina potatoes. Pickles of all kinds. All of the finny tribe; oysters and lobsters being the most dangerous. Of the meats, fresh pork and veal. Of the desserts, egg custards, pastry, cheese and preserved fruits. Of the fluids – coffee – unless ordered for medicinal purposes – raw milk, wines, ales or beers. As a matter of convenience I will introduce what in reason should constitute the proper diet for the same period of time; the modes of preparation being left to those acting as nurses. A large number of women detest gruel, or "baby-food," as they term it. In this, many, no doubt, are excusable, owing to the condition in which it may previously have been presented to them; you can make a horse leave his oats by sprinkling pepper over them. But to the point: There are about an equal number who enjoy it, and it is always best to try and avoid whims and deny one's self in every possible manner till after the milk flows freely.

A woman cannot sink on plenty of nice oat, corn-meal, or flour-gruel, minute pudding or toast panacea, given often in small quantities. Of course if any article, however well liked, is made by the gallon, so to speak, and warmed over and again, it will become to be loathed; and too great quantities taken may cause much distress in the stomach. Gruels of all kinds should be well mixed with boiling water in a clean, block tin, covered pail; then set in a clean vessel of water to boil, stirring it till well done. Coarse grain porridges should always be strained; as also should broths.

For fluids: – Shells, broma, hot milk, pure or watered to suit, are each of themselves nourishing. If the mother's milk is scant, a tea made of Indian posy or life everlasting, and drunk as table tea, with milk and sugar, if desirable, is good to increase it. The diet should become gradually solid, say in the early part of the day a broiled lamb chop, broiled beef, liver, tripe, sirloin steak, or broths without vegetables. Broiled meats retain the nutritive principles better than when otherwise cooked. If tea or coffee is found to lessen the flow of milk, it may be inferred that if continued, all of the fluids of the body will materially change.

A strict adherence to the aforesaid rules would, in a great measure, be the means of preventing cholera of infants at the breast, particularly in our crowded cities. By all means should child-bearing women eat more freely of Indian or bran bread. Brown bread can be made fresh every day where meals have to be prepared. Bread, cakes, or pastries that are puffed with soda, or whitened, or colored with any chemical substance, is not good for the health. Too much soda thins the blood; also induces baldness. Mothers of former days delighted in preparing good bread, which is the staff of life. Constipation seldom if ever troubles those that use coarse bread, and avoid much salt meat. Giving infants just a taste of every suspicious article as a sort of initiation does not always prove a sure preventive against colic. It is an old custom, and was doubtless adapted to its times and places, better knowledge, better acts. Self-denial is required of us in the Holy Writ as the only alternative, if we would be wise.

———

CHAPTER XII.

GENERAL TREATMENT OF INFANTS

CHILDREN are given to parents only for a lifetime; it may be long, or it may be very short; but to array them in fine linens, with bare neck and arms, as has been and is now to a great extent the custom in many refined communities, for public exhibition, is, it seems to me, a questionable act of parental affection. Yet many do so, and boast, when otherwise advised, of their ability to toughen. Mother, your child may be only one of a hundred to survive such experiments; ninety-nine may have been relieved by an early death.

I have looked upon the lifeless form of babes whose would-be friends had failed to toughen, but had succeeded in contributing a bud to the garden of the dead, – yea, shrouded just as they dressed them while living. Thanks to our Heavenly Father, these cruel customs are fast declining; and we may hope the day is not far distant when the feelings of the tender infants will be better protected, and their bodies covered with more comfortable material. We often see, and are expected to admire, pet dogs on the streets, covered well with cloth, though supplied with Nature's garment. Should pet Carlo die, his loss is mourned as much as that of many infants; in hundreds of cases, being borne to the cemetery followed by a number of carriages and placed in a locality adorned with monument and iron fence.

Too often babies are subjected to a variety of tortures unawares. They are expected to endure, and remain perfectly quiet, with cold food, hot food, cold air, hot air, clean clothes, dirty clothes, wet or dry clothes, thin or thick clothes, wind, dust, light or darkness, noise or quiet, scolding or-, caressing, squeezing, jolting and beating; finally they endure what no man or woman would, from one week to two years old, or till able to speak for deliverance. Previous to this time they could only squirm and kick and cry, and then, being considered sick, would be forced to take soothing drops or castor-oil. But now they can tell of their little trials by some "sound word" or striking sign. One part of the clothing of infants should not press, nor be more thickly folded, than the other. Bands and straps should be made wide and smooth. The belly-band should always be fastened on the side.

While travelling in steam-cars, coaches, etc., infants should lie down as much as possible, as sitting upright and being jostled about is liable to strain or injure for life some part of the unfinished spine; and, too, it may bring on severe vomiting and purging. When a journey is to be taken over a long route and the child is fed from a bottle, some more solid food should be substituted; as the continual re-warming of the milk, combined with the motion, renders.it unfit for nourishment. It is more frequently overfeeding and prolonged excitement that causes children to fret so when travelling, than a want of their accustomed food, A little finely-pounded, newly-corned, beef, and the compound Graham cracker, is a convenient lunch to take on a journey, especially in hot weather. This may be considered coarse fare for a babe two or three months old; but properly given, could it be so injurious as keeping them trotting, feeding on sweetened milk and water, alternating with cookies or candies which, as many can testify, is practised daily on some of our routes of travel.

As a general thing, if babes are well fed and otherwise made comfortable at every convenient interval, then allowed to lie quiet or sleep, one will need no better company on a long journey. They soon get used to changes if the change really is for their comfort.

Very young children have no more control over their eyes than they have over their lungs; and by facing an open window, as they are frequently allowed to do, often get some particle of dust in their eyes, causing them to sob and fret for miles. Should they be old enough to rub the eyes, the loving friend or guardian pronounces the cause of the suffering sleepiness, or hunger. Then comes the old bottle; if the babe doesn't drink from it, the poor little one is rolled and trotted, and sometimes slyly slapped, as a means of subduing the temper of the little . It will never do to tell what names such people call their own dear flesh and blood.

Fanning is good pastime for some women, but it is no less injurious to themselves than it is to infants, provided they apply it without regard to the condition of the body. When children are too warm their wraps should be adapted to the temperature; fanning can do more harm in a few moments, than could be repaired in a month.

A lady, going visiting with her first heir, was asked to lay off her babe's wraps. "Oh," said she, "there is no use in putting handsome wraps on baby, if I am to take them off while visiting." I may have said quite enough to prove that exposing babes to the sudden changes of temperature and atmosphere may be productive of a variety of stomach and intestinal complaints at each season of the year. Even when precaution is exercised there will be unguarded moments when the germ of disease will enter the system; but those moments should be few. I have tried to prescribe preventives as I go along which I know can be read and put up by almost any housekeeper, whether she has graduated in Chemistry or not.

Extra caution should be exercised with small children in midsummer as school vacations draw hear, as then the older children are much depended upon to care for the younger. It frequently happens that a child who has been quite thrifty begins to fall back about vacation time.

"Dog-days," they say, "give children cholera infantum," when the truth of the matter is, the accustomed food has been reduced both in quantity and quality, and they are compelled to eat or suck candies, swallow pieces of nuts, fruits, cakes, pickles, or anything the larger children choose to give. "Baby must go to ride in the carriage;" yes, and remain for hours without food, or, what is as bad, given milk to drink from a bottle that has lain beside the warm body for hours. In fact, the child thus treated may continue to pine, and really starve at the very time it should have been more lavishly fed. The system of infants has to be guarded at all times and in all places; but more especially in our New England climate, where the atmosphere is so extremely varied. Even if a child does suck the breast, it can be fed through the day, now on oatmeal and milk, and again on plain Indian meal or flour pudding. By these means, warmth is supplied to the blood, and strength to the nerves and muscles.

I hope no one will understand me as advocating heat alone as a life preserver, for I do not. It is heat alone that renders the systems of many children so susceptible to colds. It is uniformity and moderation in their whole management that I am trying to impress upon the minds of all who may desire to profit thereby.

———

CHAPTER XIII.

TIME FOR WEANING

IT IS CLAIMED, and no doubt rightfully, that it is the children of the poorer classes who suffer most in large cities from bowel complaints. To this too many are ready to say, " Amen."

But there are duties involving upon each and all, rich or poor, from which none can expect to be excused till the last known part has been performed. As the chances now appear, there need be no lack of the common comforts of life in most of our large cities and towns. This is a land of opportunities; in it the laborer gets, or should get, his hire. It therefore becomes his privilege to aid by prudence, industry, and economy, in elevating his family to the discouragement of pauperism and wilful neglect of the laws of health.'

It very often happens that those very persons, who claim to be too poor to obtain the necessary comforts of life for their little ones, will not hesitate to purchase some extortionately highpriced article, for which they must enslave themselves to pay by the week or month, and which is of far less value than their own or their children's health. I would suggest here that an extra tencent piece be deposited in safe keeping each day as a surety for a baby's comforts for the first six months; which should afterward be increased to twenty cents a day, and thus continued during its childhood.

When a child is five or six months old, it is best to begin to feed once or twice a day, so that the weaning may not be too suddenly enforced upon it. Bread, crumbled in a small quantity of milk, corn-meal pudding, mutton or chicken broth, Graham biscuit; very little salt added to the porridges is healthy. But no disagreeable substances, such as aloes, pepper or salt, should be applied to the nipples for the purpose of weaning a child; a plaster of wool or fur is more safe for the health of the child.

In this climate (Massachusetts) there are many families who fear to wean their children at any season of the year; many of them migrating from a climate less variable, and in which the customs of feeding infants are altogether different. Such mothers are deserving of no small share of sympathy. I am acquainted with hundreds of them; thank God there are some good mothers, good enough to take the blame upon themselves should their infants sicken and die after being weaned. But for all such there may be found in this little cabinet a consoling word.

Weaning is advisable before June and before December. But if a child does not thrive by reason of some constitutional weakness of the mother, it could probably rally faster by being fed otherwise, at any season of the year.

But whether a child is weakly or not it can gain nothing by continuing to suck after the ninth month; therefore, weaning is recommended about this period. If the mother breeds fast, a prolonged season of nursing but keeps her unprepared, both in strength and household matters, for the next. Then, too, it retards the healthy development of the new being, should she become pregnant while nursing. Although the mother's milk is essential to the proper growth of the child, history records evidences of noble-minded men and women who never nursed the breast, yet lived to a great age.

A great deal depends upon circumstances; for instance, it may be that even with apparently nutritive milk, the bones remain soft, the joints weak, and the flesh wastes away or remains the same. Such cases are not uncommon, especially among the very hard-working people or real indigent. Hence the necessity of seeking medical advice as to the best possible means of supplying the blood with those principles apparently lacking.

From my experience as nurse, I can say that weaning from the breast may be successfully accomplished if begun pleasantly, but decidedly, and continued. The months of May and October in the New England States are the most favorable; April and November in the Middle States, while in almost all of the Southern States weaning is advisable in March and November or December.

Waiting for a child to get all of its teeth is merely a matter of choice. Beside the inconvenience of the differences in the periods of time when the teeth get through, there is an unnecessary drain on the system of the mother, with no benefit whatever to the child.

The efforts put forth by some women to retard child-bearing is not so good as "Robbing Peter to pay Poll," because in such cases Peter is robbed, but Polly is never paid. So it seems to me that if these little ones are given in quick succession, it is just as well to have them and get through with it. Many arc the women who have borne a dozen or more children into the world, and afterwards filled positions of nobility and trust.

By taking particular notice which course is best to pursue with a child of seven or nine months, I sincerely believe the large number of infantile deaths, under one year, would be much less.

Deferring weaning for the predominance of some certain sign in the heavens, does not accord with our present progress in knowledge.

———

CHAPTER XIV.

SECTION I.
CHOLERA INFANTUM VERSUS STARVATION

IF CHOLERA of infants can be reckoned as a distinct disease, then can starvation. Whether starvation causes two-thirds of all the infantile mortalities, during the latter part of summer and the first part of autumn, or not, the symptoms indicate much the same treatment as in cholera. This statement can only be proved by close unbiased observations; books can never do it.

We will first notice some of the symptoms of starvation which may be present in real consumptive babes, also the signs of starvation that may develop in cholera; after which I shall endeavor to describe the symptoms of cholera as viewed in the light of a disease.

Starvation of a child is seldom detected by friends who may be constantly caring for it, but the eye of a practitioner cannot fail to do so at once, assisted by the required information. Notwithstanding, a physician may permit doubts to enter the mind, or through over cautiousness conceal the real opinion.

SIGNS OF STARVATION

A child may be apparently well and hearty at birth, may thrive even at the breast for a few months; then all at once seem to fail. It may be fed on whatever is ordered if not at the breast from the first; yet barely live on for months, whining, drooping, and struggling, as it were, to live. Such patients lay awake, listen, and watch the motion of passing objects; when spoken to, will try to indicate something, look pitiful, act intelligent concerning wearing apparel or toys. In fact such a child is termed cross. It will cry after everything it sees, and that it don't see; will slap things, such as cake or crackers, out of your hand. Nothing offered is welcomed as a relish. The bowels are generally loose, the urine copious; yet in many cases the water is voided in large quantities, while the bowels are dry. The eyes retain their brightness, as if to invite attention to the fact, " I would thrive if I had what I need." The patient may drink half a gallon a day without the least sign of satisfaction.

Starvation may begin with the fetal development either from lack of nourishment from the system of the parent, or by reason of repeated attempts at abortion; either of which is sufficient to blunt the vitality of the germ. Such children are likely to "hang on," perhaps till the period of youth, and with good care may arrive to manhood or womanhood. The most doubtful cases are those that have a dry cough, eat a great deal, yet are never content, bloat at certain times, and grow more stupid; the body becoming a mere skeleton, and with difficulty kept warm. The new being is dependent upon the state of the parent's blood from the moment of conception till weaned from the breast. If the food upon which a child is fed is the cause of the trouble, it should be changed as soon as possible. If from other causes there are medicines which can in a measure supply the needed basis. But generally the real cause is not known or even suspected until too late to repair the injury, and the patient dies after having exhibited all signs of consumption. Children born of consumptive parents may come out quite bright in some branches of thought, yet be quite delicate, seldom passing the flower of youth in life.

I feel incompetent to decide whether a consumptive mother had better nurse her child, and thus fasten the germ of disease upon it, with a view to prolonging her own life; or whether it is best for her to yield to her fate, and substitute some different food for the chance of her child's life.

SECTION II.
SYMPTOMS OF EMPTINESS OR STARVATION, WHICH MAY LEAD TO CHOLERA

If, as heretofore mentioned, the solid or nutritive principle of the milk has been withheld from the babe by adulteration in any way, the blood becomes watery, the fat cells cannot develop, the tissues that hold the fluid with which to moisten the parts dries away, and the flesh becomes soft or skinny. The milk may be nutritive, too, and yet for some reason fail to mix with the juices in the stomach so as to insure healthy blood.

These facts, however, are seldom found out by a casual medical attendant until the powers of digestion are too weak to derive much benefit from an other kind of diet. Besides, the expense of the articles mostly ordered by physicians renders a trial almost out of the question. There are, however, many articles of nourishment obtainable, which, if perseveringly administered, will do much to assist in building up the little frame.

The most marked of the signs that may end in cholera are vomiting, dullness of the eyes, rolling the head, as if to rock, spitefully crying when taken up to be changed, and begging for everything, as they say; also crying, if old enough, for the very things no one thinks it should have. If a child could have some of what it smells and craves, at such times, no doubt but that recovery would commence. But a general languidness of the whole system, and a loathing of the sight of a bottle or its accustomed food, shows signs of certain destruction. In the last stage the child screams faintly, starts at the sound of almost anything; sometimes the breathing is scarcely perceptible. The discharges from the bowels are seldom white and frothy, as in the last stage of acute cholera; owing, perhaps, to the fact that the diet has been continued in the former, whereas in the latter all food is generally suspended during treatment, except it be fluids of the mildest nature; unlike in the last stage of consumption, when the little sufferer seems to watch every movement of its nearest friend, sometimes rising half way up to look about, then falling back exhausted, it now lies quiet.

It may be remarked just here that infants affected with inanition or starvation, consumption and cholera, most invariably retain to the last hour their instinct to suck, whether it be of the bottle or of the breast It is a well-known fact that infants who were nearly destroyed by starvation from being fed on poor milk by hand, have been successfully raised by being put on breast-milk.

SECTION III.
CHOLERA INFANTUM - INFANTILE CHOLERA

We will now consider that much-dreaded disease termed "cholera infantum." I have seen babes attacked with it from two weeks old and upwards. A child may be nursing at the breast or feeding from a bottle, when all of a sudden it leaves off, and looks languidly about in a comparatively stupid and pitiful manner; the eyes lose their lustre, are rolled about as if not noticing any particular object. Fluids are thrown up as soon as swallowed; passages from the bowels are frequent, though many times but a speck in the centre of a wet napkin, most of the report being wind. The matter discharged at first is likely to show in some measure the cause of the irritation.

After the acidity has been corrected by medicines, unlike a simple looseness, the purging and vomiting of infantile cholera still continue, showing conclusively the inactivity of the internal organs of digestion. In some cases the remedies that are scientifically administered pass out into the napkin unchanged; in others, they seem to lodge somewhere and dry up. The chances are always considered favorable to recovery if the remedies have a desirable action.

A child may drool or throw up its food at any time, yet be quite healthy. If a babe is sucking, and the mother indulges in a mixed or meat and vegetable diet too early, the first passages after it is taken sick will show signs of heat, fermentation and inflammation; they will either be of a deep yellow, or more or less green, and slimy. In such instances it is always advisable to take the infant from the breast for a while and feed it on arrow-root boiled in water, till the acidity is corrected; then in milk, no sugar being added, alternating with gum-arabic water. The mother, or wet-nurse, having been put under strict diet for a week, might with propriety resume nursing. Robust, perfectly developed children are apt to exhibit considerable vitality through the different phases of the disease; but as far as my experience has been, they succumb to the worst more quickly than the more delicate-appearing.

As the disease progresses the little sufferer will thrust its fingers in its mouth, as if to intimate hunger or dryness, and gag, as though something was sticking in the throat. The hands and arms are the most active. The lower extremities are seldom moved from one position; and when moved by any one, they are quickly reversed. Every movement of the body, in bathing or changing, is followed by a discharge from the bowels. These discharges vary in consistence even before any medicine has been given. After the bowels have been purged, as is recommended by most physicians to begin with, the discharges from the bowels may run off frequently, and in small quantities, depositing in the napkin a whitish, frothy fluid, which settles down to a chalky substance, giving out the smell of lime. If such emissions continue, they will effect a rapid destruction; or they may have the same appearance from the beginning if the internal organs have been previously rendered weak from starvation, or rather where the food has been but little better than water sweetened; and, too, these frothy emissions greatly chafe the parts if they are allowed to remain soiled.

The tongue is dry and stiff, as a general thing, throughout the disease. The body, with the exception of the belly, is dry and cool. The mouth is apt to be hot from the beginning, a sign remarked by mothers who have suckled babes with cholera; in the last stage, the disposition to sleep, but start at the least noise; the mouth lying half open, the intelligent attempts to suck; the decrease of the discharges from the bowels; the cessation of retching; the sinking in of the features; the nervous grasping, as if to catch some passing object; jerking of the body, and moaning, may be looked upon as unfavorable signs.

It is a great mistake to conclude that infants will have cholera if weaned early, or if they are to be artificially nursed. The fear comes from persons having been so educated within the last half century.

All kinds of preparations are advertised and eagerly sought for baby diet; as if the internal organs of babes were entirely different from what they were before, and must needs be supplied with something more supernatural than those of the adult. The symptoms of cholera are by no means uniform. For instance, they may be cut short, or aggravated by overdosing, before the facts in the case are made known. Thus, if paregoric, laudanum, or any alcoholic carminatives are habitually put in the drink, the most marked signs will be the smell of the breath, the presence of constipation, stupor and sinking in of the features more or less, with very little vomiting. Such cases, no doubt, are seldom admitted, the victims being dead, or nearly so, when medical aid is called.

SECTION IV.
GENERAL TREATMENT OF CHOLERA INFANTUM, MEDICAL AND DOMESTIC

Unfortunately for many children, it is usually in the last stage of the disease that a physician is consulted. Probably any number of palliatives have been given with good intentions and high hopes of success. For one, the old cleaning-out remedy, so much thought of by old ladies, and doctors not a few, – castor-oil. Whatever may be deemed as proper treatment, it should be remembered that nothing short of the most untiring vigilance on the part of the attendant, guided by Divine aid, can bring success in raising a child on whom cholera has fastened its blighting fangs. Yet what encouragement it is to know that by those means it can be saved.

My course for the last fifteen years has been to first ascertain, if possible, the cause of cholera, and have it removed; also particularly to inquire how long it has been since the child has been noticed to fail in the effort to suck; then as to the color and frequency of the discharges. I have never known, through my observations of over twentythree years, any better corrector of acidity, sourness in the human bowels, than calcined magnesia.

After giving from two to three grains every hour, or according to the degree of acidity, until it is all apparently changed, then, as cautiously as needful, I proceed to quiet the motion of the bowels, as in case of purging within the month, by the use of mixture No. i, which ii put up by a regular chemist, and given according to directions, can be no more objectionable because inserted in this little book than thousands of other recipes scattered over the community by tons in expensive books.

No. I, R. Mixtura Creatae, preperata, zj. – Chalk Mixture, Aquae Cinnam. zss. – Cinnamon Water. Add Opii Tinct. Gutta vj. – Laudanum.

Shake well before using. Dose – A small teaspoonful after each stool. Increase the dose according to age of patient. Of course it is not expected that the inexperienced would attempt to administer anything other than domestic remedies, unless put up according to the rules of art.

For a decided case of cholera, it is best to begin with half a teaspoonful of the mixture; which, by the by, should be sucked down by the patient very slowly, in order to have it remain on the stomach. No time should be wasted listening to the old story of working off a bowel complaint; few are the adults that ever have survived the experiment, much less the weakly infant. Deaths from cholera cannot possibly be so numerous in consequence of the discharges having been checked too soon, for the usual precaution is not to arrest them; so they are let to go on increasing, till all hopes of contracting the vessels are vain. It would be well in all cases before administering Mixture No. I, to fill a flannel bag with hops, wring it out of warm, salt water and lay it over the chest and belly, re-wetting every two hours; this done will alone sometimes prove successful.

When the mouth remains dry and hot, a little cool water, sucked slowly from a spoon, does seem to revive the little sufferer, and I have no reason to doubt its efficacy in abating the suffering, if not the disease. Stimulant astringents are what is needed after the passages are checked. The least mite of Nature's stimulant – common salt – laid on the back part of the tongue, will excite a flow of saliva, and greatly assist in removing a sort of hair-worm which has been noticed to infest the throat in some patients. When there is a continuance of vitality, and the passages continue to be green, or tinged with blood, and external cooling applications, as of flaxseed poultices, have been well tried, an effort should be made to stimulate the liver; this is very likely to be the case where the age and constitution of the child is sufficient to permit the disease to run on for quite a while. Hydrargium chloridum-calomel, is sometimes the most reliable drug that can be used to correct that. This drug is unsafe in the hands of the inexperienced, but quick and safe when under the guidance of medical skill. The dose for a child six months old should never exceed one-sixteenth of a grain, or one grain in sixteen hours, followed by a sip of warm milk.

The nourishment during this time should consist of the breast-milk, if possible; if not, arrowroot boiled in milk and gum water, fed from a spoon twice a day, or oftener. But either should always be given about a half hour after any medicine, unless otherwise directed. Cold water should never be allowed to a patient while medicine is being administered, the nature of which is unknown. Light, air, sponging the body with warm salt water, a change of clothing or bedding, each tends to stimulate the pores, quench thirst, and give tone to the whole system. Thin flourgruel acts as a pasty lining to the entrails. After the irritation has ceased, great care is required to prevent a relapse; therefore in all cases when the breast-milk cannot be obtained, the various vegetable astringents should be relied on to build up the muscles, the different grains, as cornmeal, starch and oatmeal, given often but in small quantities, will build up the fat cells. If, after the liver has been acted upon, the green stools do not cease, and there seem to be a general weakness of the digestive organs, the juice of the blackberry, raspberry, or whortleberry, will, in most cases, effect a cure; also, the rinds of ripe peaches boiled in milk till well done, strained, and given when cool – a teaspoonful five or six times during the day, and about as often at night – is excellent. The effect of either of these remedies should be closely watched, as by their astringent nature they might induce constipation.

With a view to the comfort of the sick one, and the convenience of the nurse, it is better to prepare a bed of some light material, on which the patient can lie with its body flexed. Too often the little creature is forced to lie in a narrow place, or more frequently on the lap, in one position, till it would seem as if it would be paralyzed. There should be two sets of bedding in order to expedite recovery. The material should consist of goods that could be easily washed, and kept clean. It is essential, too, that flannel be worn by the sick one; but it is a sad mistake to imagine that flannel clothes do not need changing as often as cotton ones.

When I have suggested a bed for sick infants, some grandmas have thought me cruel. But in such critical cases as the one in question, a few moments' trotting and rolling on the lap might undo all that it had taken weeks to do. Should the stomach become settled, but the lower bowels remain rather weak and liable to looseness, and there is no fever present, I think much of the burnt brandy in small doses. I prepare it in the following manner: Take a wineglassful of the best brandy, one tablespoonful of refined sugar, dissolve it well, then pour it in a shallow dish and set fire to it with a lighted paper, not a match; when the blue flame is off it is fit for use, and should be put in a clean vial and labelled. Of this, I give to a child six weeks old and upward, six drops in a little water, say about three times within twelve hours. To one six months and upward, I give ten to fifteen drops twice a day. This warms up the stomach and stimulates the digestive fluid glands to action. After the brandy has had the desired effect, a speedy recovery may be hoped for. The bathing, nourishing diet, quietness, and, above all, patience, need to be continued with greater zeal when recovery is apparent. The recovery from cholera is probable only when the surroundings are favorable; it is doubtful where the locality is densely inhabited, the disease prevalent, and where there is a lack of means to provide ample care and nourishment. Patients recovering from a disease like cholera, which so undermines the nervous system, require a deal of determination to 'prevent the undoing of what has been done by catering to their whims.

———————

CHAPTER XV.

THE CAUSES AND PREVENTION OF CHOLERA INFANTUM

IT HAS been argued, authoritatively, no doubt, that the causes of cholera infantum are, poor milk, bad air arising from old water-soaked cellars, of tenement houses, or when it affects those of all conditions in life, the rich, the poor, the black and the white, – its cause is said to be in some atmospherical phenomena. I think the last mentioned might be reconsidered, since it appears, from noticing the health records, that mortalities from this disease have increased in extremely warm weather only in proportion to the influx of emigrants.

If poor or adulterated milk were the cause, there should be an entire absence of the disease at present, since such stringent efforts are now put forth to punish the wretch who dares adulterate the milk he sells.

Quite enough has been published of late concerning the adulteration of milk by putting in saltpetre, chalk, glucose, anotta, and other ingredients for the purpose of increasing the density, while water is added to increase the quantity. Admitting these shameful facts, have they not been practised long enough for the news to have reached the ears of every housewife in America? Why, I have been hearing those reports at different times for forty years. With these facts, then, so generally known, why do people water the milk they buy, and depend on it for the support and nourishment of infants? There is trouble somewhere. Children have been successfully raised on milk from animals, both in city and country, at all seasons of the year, in hot or cold climates; and many thousands of aged mothers to-day, could doubtless advise young women in the matter of baby raising, did they not settle down in the thought that the young people are getting all such knowledge along with their great facilities for education. Oh, how sadly mistaken have many thousands gone to their long home!

The management of cholera infantum is not to be coveted; the best of all is to know how to prevent it. I sincerely believe that the greater number of cases of cholera are induced by the unnatural custom of preparing a bottle of food, and putting the child in a position to sleep while it sucks from it. Where is the woman or man who can sleep and eat at the same time The mode of preparing it is generally putting a little milk with a quantity of water, and a little sugar, into a half -pint bottle – if the babe is only a few days old – and this is kept close to its warm body for hours, or what is just as bad, re-warmed every time it is suspected that the baby is hungry.

Pure milk needs no watering; it is simply converted into slops by so doing. It contains naturally sugar, butter, lime, and all that is required for the nourishment of the young.

The saliva of the glands of the mouth and the juices of the stomach are as fully able to dilute and separate the life principles of milk for a babe, as they are to prepare solid food for the maintenance of the adult. We eat a beefsteak in its purity, risking the after effects; were there more ventures in administering pure food to helpless infants, no doubt but there would soon appear a change in the physique of our young men and women.

To insure a healthy meal, an infant should invariably be fed with care before laying it down from the very first day of its attempt to suck from a bottle, for the following reasons: – As the babe dozes, its breath goes down the tube; the heat and churning motion together separate the butter globules from the fluid so that they cannot get through the holes, unless, as is often the case, the holes are made too large, for some selfish convenience. And by this latter means the danger of strangulation becomes more imminent if the child is left alone. Scores of times have I seen the infant tugging away between naps, for hours, trying to get what it should have finished in less than twenty or thirty minutes, and been sleeping soundly.

Numbers of them cry half the night, or are pacified by having the rubber nipple of a filthysmelling sucking-bottle continually stuck in the mouth. Thus some babes are literally worn out sucking, trying to get a bare subsistence. Even if an infant nurses from the breast, it is wrong to put off suckling it till the powers are almost overcome by sleep. While we are aware that its breath cannot go into the mamma, the liability to strangulation is none the less apparent.

There can be no more important duties to perform in the capacity of housekeeping than that of caring for the helpless babe. Women doctors, or, more properly speaking, doctresses of medicine, although usually treated with less courtesy by doctors, are, nevertheless, by them considered to be in their proper sphere in the confinement-room and nursery. While I feel under no obligations to them for their charity, I must admit their honesty and truthfulness in the matter; for surely woman cannot fill a single position in the world so freighted with material, out of which the moral and physical condition of humanity can be affected either for good or evil.

———

CHAPTER XVI.

CONVENIENT METHODS FOR RAISING INFANTS WITHOUT THE BREAST

A SMALL bottle holding an ounce, for the first, should be in readiness; a smooth round hole made in the cork, through which to put a quill; the whole to be well covered with a strong soft linen, the edges of which should be hemmed and securely tied under the lip of the bottle. This constituted a sucking-bottle of fifty years ago. The modern rubber tube and nipple, if composed of healthy material, removed from the mouth and washed as soon as possible after using, may do as well. If a child is allowed to sleep all it naturally inclines to, four ounces of milk or two of cream will suffice it during the day, say from seven or eight o'clock in the morning until six in the evening. From that time until bed-time, say nine or ten o'clock, half as much. After ten, the feeding should be as seldom as will allow of comfort. In this way, one pint of milk or half a pint of pure cream will be sufficient to last a babe of from one to four weeks old, a whole day, allowing the cream to be increased to nearly a pint by watering. The quantity should be increased gradually, while the number of meals during the night should decrease. By these means a babe will soon cease to be any trouble after bed hours. Only remember that it has nerves, through which it is supplied with feelings.

A small bottle insures renewal of the food, for positively the same milk that a child has tried to draw from a bottle for any length of time is not fit to be re-warmed or offered to it again; and if persisted in, will act as a slow poison, which may develop into cholera at any period of infantile existence. Again, if milk flows evenly, the butter globules do not form in the bottle. If the milk flows too fast into the child's mouth, the healthful benefits of a meal is lost.

I have often seen mothers force, with apparent anger, great spoonfuls down the throats of their babes; perhaps such would think this cruel if done by a nurse or overburdened servant-girl.

If a child has cold in the head, so that the nostrils are stopped, means should be used at once to clear them. No one can swallow properly with the nostrils stopped up. To remove the cause daily will prevent those sickening accumulations. A strict attention to cleanliness, and frequent applications of sweet oil, or lard, or goose oil, with a feather, is all that is wanting to prevent so many cases of sore noses, terminating in the entire loss of smell, and not infrequently the destruction of the soft bones of the nose, or even the cause of cancer. Feeding during the night should be discontinued as soon as possible, as it is then that mistakes of giving the food too hot or too cold are liable to occur. Night feeding may only be avoided by encouraging babes to keep awake during the evening. But if they must be put to sleep early in the evening, as a rule, to suit some one's convenience, it may be expected that, as a rule, they will wake up just when other people are sleepy, and desire some notice. Infants from three months old and upward will thrive well on a pint and a half of milk a day, but will get on much faster if fed with rolled compound cracker and milk during the day. It is needful to give some babes fluids only, while others starve on them. It is the continual emptiness that causes many children to fret and whine; for whatever they smell, cooking excites their appetites more or less as they grow in intelligence. And, too, children take appetites from their parents in a marked degree. As a doctress, I never could feel it justifiable to direct any woman to wean her babe on account of any conceited inability on her part to suckle it.

I knew a lady whose infant of two weeks was taken suddenly ill while nursing. A doctor was sent for, and when he was informed by the mother that her milk was too rich for the babe, he at once advised her to wean it. What more, think you, could have been expected with a diet of soft boiled eggs for breakfast, custards for dinner, and wines or ales at night? Surely if women ask no questions of the doctors, no answers can be given. It does seem too bad to punish the child for the faults of the parent. Eggs, like fish, may act like sure poison to the milk of a nursing woman. The continued dry belly-ache or wind colic so much fretted over by old ladies in the past, was but a sequence of the custom of feeding lying-in women on wine custards. During the time of those baby afflictions it seldom entered the mind of either nurse or doctor what caused the almost universal three months' "belly-ache" of infants. Articles that may not perceptibly affect the mother or wetnurse, as the case may be, may prove certain death to the sucking babe.

Infants should never be obliged to lie over their accustomed hours of rising. If necessity demands this, however, there can be far more gained by taking up, cleaning, exercising, and giving them a fresh supply of food. It is not that too much sleep may be enjoyed, but that the condition in which it is taken should warrant the refreshment needed to build up the new being.

Soft bones, enlarged joints, inverted feet, flattened back-heads, sickening sores, dropsy, blindness, and numerous ills have befallen infants from the thoughtless practice of letting them lie too much in soiled clothes, and being insufficiently fed. In the matter of early rising, the farmer's child has the advantage of the city child. In the country a babe is looked upon as one of the family, with rights that men are bound to respect; but in the city it is, "Wait dear, till Johnny comes home from school."

There may appear small white scales or patches on the tongue and inner surface of the mouth. This is commonly called "thrush." It is usually caused by too great heat, either of surroundings or diet. Sugar in large quantities will create it in some babes. This complaint *may* run on to an alarming extent, but yields readily to mild treatment timely applied. It not infrequently happens that, during the presence of apthae in the mouth, the back passage becomes sore, or presents much the same appearance. The thrush is then said by old ladies to have gone through the child's bowels. This can hardly be a fact, since the whole trouble disappears readily upon removing the cause.

I have seen it upon the edges and under-surface of the eyelids, in babes that are allowed to sleep where it is generally very close, with the face covered over, or closely nestled to the breast of the mother. The treatment should be cooling. Calcined magnesia in from three to five-grain doses daily, for a week or two, and gently washing the scales over once a day with sugar and water, will, if persisted in, effect a cure. Giving "baby just a taste of everything mamma eats," is no doubt a frequent cause of this distressing complaint.

If the appetite fails in a child, and there is no perceptible cause, and the mouth is dry and hot for a time, it will do no harm to touch the front edge of the tongue with a mite of table-salt. One or two trials will suffice to set the saliva flowing, then with a little coaxing and proper food the appetite will return. I may have digressed somewhat, but as aptha; is frequently accompanied by diarrhea, I deem it well to guard against fear and loss of hope that might ensue from its being mistaken for cholera. In any case of vomiting or purging of infants, great caution is required not to give all kinds of palliative suggested by incomers; this is "going it blind," so to speak. Cholera is a terrible disease, and should be subdued as speedily as possible. At best it leaves its merciless traces throughout the remainder of life; the victim being frequently annoyed by choleric pains, indigestion, nervousness and cough. To sum up all, the causes of cholera infantum are movable unless fixed by some perceptible atmospherical pressure. The causes of cholera are no doubt overlooked by the major portion of a community where its ravages from time to time have been the greatest, and consequently no efforts are put forth in a general way to prevent a repetition of its visits. Even where the conditions of the atmosphere may give rise to cholera, its force can be modified, and the number of fatalities lessened. I have frequently been asked if cholera is contagious; in answer, I can safely say, it is not, as a disease; but like causes will produce like effects, in the same locality, and at the same time. In regard to the fumes of carbolic acid, chloride of lime, sulphur, and the like, as disinfectants, I believe that they are all decidedly depressing, and against the speedy recovery of cholera patients if used in immediate contact. The removal from a crowded district in time of an apparent epidemic is decidedly commendable. It is well known that poverty, wretchedness, and crime favor an increase of mortality from this disease. Yet the prospects of thousands remain the same year after year.

Strange 'tis, but true; in all this vast American domain, is there not room for the welfare of God's moving images? In the city of Richmond, Va., the heat is much more constant in midsummer than in Boston, Mass. Yet of the three hundred visits among the most forsaken poor of the former city, infantile cholera is comparatively rare, and from July 15, 1877, to Oct. 30, of the same year, I found but one case of cholera from starvation; that being a case where the parent had to be out all day, while it fed from a bottle or sucked on something. Whatever saved many others in like situation, it is beyond my power to tell. There would no doubt be more numerous fatalities with children in warm climates if it was the almost universal custom to feed them on slops; but on the contrary, where they are not at the breast, among the laboring classes at least, they are fed on what is convenient for the rest of the family; and although many times the fare is decidedly objectionable, the Lord crowns the efforts for good with success.

Going South, as I did, a teetotaller, I was pleasantly surprised to find that the freed people were no more intemperate than any other would be if placed in like circumstances; perhaps not so much so as many of those who could better understand how, when freedom came, all of the necessaries of life were speedily cut off from them, but where rum and ruin were, they could find an open door. Instead of setting out a decanter and glasses, as was the custom in the days of slavery (according to all accounts), I noticed a delicacy, lest they might be suspected of wrong-doing. In order to encourage the impression for reform, whenever an opportunity offered, I would say that children have grown weaker every generation in families that have indulged in the use of rum and tobacco.

Frugality is advisable; looking to securing a home in the outer limits, away from all objectionable odors, where rooms can be ventilated and sunned in winter as well as in summer. Every room in a dwelling should be swept and dusted' once or twice a week, the beds aired, and bedding changed. The general custom of housekeepers in our large and crowded cities, of keeping their rooms dark, winter or summer, inoculates into the system the germs of more diseases than could be enumerated and prescribed for in a day. A cheerful home with a small tract of land in the country, with wholesome food and water, is worth more to preserve health and life, than a house in a crowded city with luxuries and twenty rooms to let. That bad air is not the sole cause of infantile cholera, I will mention an incident in proof. While travelling through some of the thinly-settled districts of the British Provinces during the prevalence of cholera in the autumn of 1865, I noticed that most of the children suffering from the disease were those of parents whose circumstances would not warrant the comforts of life. This was during the months of September and October, when fish, oysters, milk and eggs are indulged in to some extent. I thought the custom of advising the removal of such patients to some elevated point near the salt sea air could avail but little, since they were near the sea-air and mostly in well-ventilated houses, judging from the style of architecture. Also I noticed the same uncertainty on the part of women as to the management of the complaint as in the States. Herb teas, no matter what their nature, "catnip tea, castor -oil and paregoric." Every drink sweetened, as a rule. The visits of the doctor few and far between; " so many cases he can't possibly get around to them all." I had a little charge at the time whom I never left an hour from the time it was taken ill till its recovery, three weeks later. The family doctor called in occasionally, but the circumstances of the young parents were such as to warrant the necessary aids to a recovery which it was my good fortune to administer. This was in a thickly-settled locality in the city of St. John, N. B., while in many upland towns of Nova Scotia it generally proved fatal. May we not be too willing to agree in charging our Heavenly Father with poisoning the air, so that it destroys infants by the tens of thousands in less than a quarter of a century?

Let the interested humanitarian visit those families where necessity demands the absence of the parent a part or all of each day, to seek a daily subsistence, leaving the youngest to the care of the eldest, winter or summer, before deciding whether it is a want of stamina, the depressions of the atmosphere, or indirect starvation which causes so great infantile mortality at certain seasons of the year. It is a mistake to suppose that cold milk given to a babe in excessive hot weather will answer as well as if warmed. The human stomach is supplied with heat from the blood and natural fluids, and when a quantity of anything colder than the contents of the organ is poured into it, the process needful to a healthy digestion cannot go on properly.

CHAPTER XVII.

SECTION I.
TEETHING MADE EASY

AS A GENERAL THING, children begin to get teeth from the ages of five to seven months. The middle, or incisors, in the lower jaw, are the first to appear, one in advance of the other; and, too, these may get through almost unnoticed. It is a custom with many persons to begin poking into a babe's mouth just as soon as it shows restlessness, or signs of getting teeth; and, perceiving that it bites, as naturally it should, they at once introduce a rubber, or some kind of hard substance, for it to bite upon, to assist the teeth through. This is unnatural, and liable to increase the already feverish and fretful condition of the child. The more artificial friction is applied, the more inflamed will the gums become. Teaching babes to bite on the fingers, rings, dolls, and the like, is but subjecting them to torture which they would gladly repel could they speak.

There is really no set time at which babes should get teeth; some begin much younger than others. There are instances recorded of children being born with teeth; this, however, is of rare occurrence; but it is a common thing to see the forms of well-developed teeth through the delicate, transparent cover of the gums at birth. The development of these little bones is really peculiar, and worthy of the most profound study; but I shall only attempt to speak here in reference to the maturing process, or their making ready to come through the gums, hoping, by so doing, much of the seeming anxiety of young mothers and nurses from this cause may be removed.

The term "critical period" is applied so much to the process of getting teeth that it becomes fixed upon the heart of many mothers long before its time of beginning. The most that must be guarded against is fatigue, either from lying or sitting too long in one position, irregular habits of feeding, and untidyness. The more a child slavers when getting teeth, the better; yet this is not always a sign of coming teeth. The slaver, nevertheless, keeps the mouth cool and moist, preventing dry or papular eruptions. Cold water is advisable, given frequently from a spoon, while the teeth are breaking through. If the child is at the breast, well; if not, its food should consist of scalded milk; as it grows in strength, oatmeal is a good addition. If hearty and craving in disposition, Graham crackers crumbled in and fed to it with a spoon, about twice a day, generally gives due satisfaction If the passes from the bowels are numerous, yet healthy, a drink of gum-arabic water two or three times a day, together with flour added to the milk in place of oatmeal, will generally regulate them. Over distention of the stomach by sweetened drinks should be strictly avoided. The extreme fretfulness of the babe at this time is caused by the pressure of the crown of the tooth against the sore or swollen gum. When the teeth get through, the cause of the distress will be removed. Should the gums continue painful, as is often the case with the double teeth, a dentist or the family physician should be consulted at once; and, if Nature has made ready the bony structure to be bared, the least touch with the lancet will part the skin and assist it through. I repeat that the gums in a healthy condition seldom need lancing; they may be left to Nature. Admitting, however, that there are numerous cases of daily occurrence where the lancet ought to be applied, it is positively forbidden by some would-be friend. The surest way to stop toothache in the adult is to extract the decayed member, and so the surest way to cut short the sufferings of an innocent babe, whose gums are swollen and painful, is to lance the gum, and let the tooth come through. Children whose mouths are dry from being kept too hot, eating highly-seasoned or salt food, or from some hereditary disposition, are especially liable to be late getting teeth, and there are many living evidences where none ever appeared.

The greater mischief is done to the whole nervous system by the unnatural but ancient custom of pressing and rubbing the gum long before, or at the time the teeth are making ready to come through. I believe it possible to trace the cause of insanity to the pernicious custom of rubbing the gums of infants. Once commenced, it, like all applications that arouse the feelings, is looked for at a certain time, rendering the child a burden rather than a pleasure to the family circle. It is strange, but true, that the anxiety of some mothers to see the much-mooted "critical period" culminates in a desire to bring it about.

SECTION II.
THE ORDER IN WHICH THE TEETH COME

The four cutters may appear in the upper jaw before the lower ones; two may come close together, then the two lower ones. After a while, the other cutters get through, making eight in all, – four up and four down. Then comes the canine or dog teeth, of which there are four, – two upper and two lower. About this time the stomach begins to be more or less affected, according to the surroundings; the child is said to be "cutting its eyeteeth." Lastly come the grinders, of which there are eight, – four upper and four lower, – twenty in all, – and are denominated milk teeth. The following is the order in which they appear: Eight incisors or cutting teeth; four canine or dog teeth; eight molars or grinders.

Many babes keep their mouths firmly shut against rubbing intruders, and, as if to surprise one, open the mouth to cry, and display quite a row of pearly teeth. Healthy, well-developed children generally have all their first teeth by the third year. Backward or rachitic children often have none at that age. I am acquainted with several apparently robust persons who never had all of their first teeth, and who are now probably past the age to get them.

After the first teeth are through, precaution is necessary to preserve them. They should be kindly looked after each day, any foreign particles removed, and the teeth wiped with a wet cloth. No hot or exceedingly cold, sour, hard, or brittle substances should be allowed to be bitten on, as they are easily broken. A snagged-tooth child looks almost as repulsive as a snagged-tooth man or woman. If people will let their children go around, as in midsummer they frequently do, with bare feet on the cold sidewalk, or with wet feet from having waded in every accessible puddle of water, while getting their grinders, they should not wonder at the great number of deaths under four years old. For thus many, besides suffering greatly with pain from teething, take cold, which may develop in lung fever. Hardly any one says, "My child died from exposure while teething." Nay, but pneumonia sets in, and the teething has to bear the blame. The primary cause is overshadowed by the probable secondary cause of death. If the first teeth are well cared for, all decaying ones removed in good season, the foundation of a handsome, permanent set will be sure, there being no constitutional diseases of the teeth themselves.

Loose, aching teeth are no less annoying to children than to adults, and it is cruel to force them to endure the pain when a few cents paid out to a dentist would remove it at once. Uneven, overlapped, inverted, projecting, and anomalous teeth are nearly all occasioned by neglecting to remove the milk teeth in proper time. Usually the application of the dental forceps is no more dreaded than the linen thread.

It is a mistake to suppose that children must have sore ears, eyes, mouth, nose, head, or some sickening eruption of the skin while teething. On the contrary, it has been clearly proved that too much heat and uncleanliness are the chief causes of these repulsive troubles. If sores or pimples do appear at times, they can with propriety be washed often with warm water, anointed with cold cream, till well; or, if there are bleeding pimples, sprinkling the parts, after washing each day, with calcined magnesia and elm flour, in equal quantities, will soon effect a cure. Babes whose scalps are well cleaned at birth seldom, if ever, have sore head. There is not the slightest danger of giving: the child cold by cleaning it off as fast as possible, when discovered. I have frequently seen little three-year-old ones playing about with not only a sore patch full of greasy dirt on their scalp, but a filthy-looking cap, called a tar cap; in this way they have been kept till the hair tubes were as completely destroyed as if the head had been scalded. It is not very encouraging to know that the great wisdom which prompts people to do, or persist in having done, these mischievous things, is never sufficient to find the remedy for the injury done. Whenever scurf does form on the head, it may be removed by applying sweet oil; should there be disposition to matter, a wash, made by boiling burdock root in water, – say half an ounce to a pint, – applied once or twice a day, is cleansing. To heal a healthy scalp sore, red oak bark, steeped in water, – sayh alf an ounce to a quart, – makes a good wash. Sometimes the cure is very tedious; but, with due patience, all will be well.

When children get so that they can nibble, it is not a good plan to begin putting candies and knickknacks in their hands as a play-rule; for this habit induces, to a certainty, all the unpleasant symptoms attendant upon indigestion; the most marked of which, in children, is unrest, fretfulness, loss of eye-sight, loss of teeth, and dwarfed statures. I take pleasure in recommending the following as a healthy, desirable kind of biscuit for children: Take one teacupful each of wheat and Graham or

Indian corn-meal; one-half cup of brown sugar or molasses; half teaspoonful of salt; mix with warm milk, knead well, cut into medium size cracker form, and bake quickly. They are nice, and should be eaten at regular meal times, dry, or crumbed in milk-and-water tea. Milk should never be withheld from children on a pretext of being feverish.

———

CHAPTER XVIII.

COMPLICATIONS OF TEETHING WITH DISEASES

DIARRHEA is the most common trouble during the teething period, and is deserving of the most generous treatment. Should the food seem to disturb the stomach and pass away undigested, or in pieces, with some degree of sourness, the pulverized magnesia in from three to five -grain doses, once or twice a day, will correct it; after which gum-water, or milk, made like gruel, with' flour, should be the chief diet till relieved. No fresh fish or eggs should be allowed in time of diarrhea. Should the discharges continue, frequent drinks of a decoction of blackberry or raspberry leaves, or what is just as well, the juice of those ripe fruits, may be given in spoonful-doses. Also the fine lean corned beef, rolled or pounded fine and fed slowly in small quantities – say a tablespoonful during the day – will frequently arrest the whole trouble; emptiness, it will be remembered being an exciting cause of diarrhea as much as overfeeding. There will be emptiness if a continual nibbling is allowed, with the smallest chance of ever getting a substantial meal. Usually, in the diarrhea of teething, there is great thirst, which may best be abated by giving plentifully of thin, cool gum-arabic water, no sugar. It is this everlasting sugar sweetening that creates fermentation at such times. It is the over-indulgence in objectionable food that causes much of the bowel complaint in teething, rather than the teething itself. We are aware that the pain caused by a coming tooth is annoying, yet this is no reason why children cannot be kindly prohibited from grasping and tasting everything they seem to see or cry for. Children are very sensitive to odors, therefore cooking and eating should be done as remote from them as possible. In this matter, however, many of the laboring classes and indigent are deserving of sympathy; being either from choice, or ill-fortune, huddled together in close tenements, where each can smell what the other is cooking. And it is next to impossible for them to better the future condition or prospects of their offspring while continuing to live so. It may not be unprofitable to insert here what I have frequently suggested as a sanitary measure : that is, for families to make it a rule not to occupy the last room at the top of the house, even for storing goods; as carpets, trunks, hanging garments or curtains, and bedding catch and retain the odors ascending from below. Smoke, gases, dusts, breaths of inmates, steam, the odors arising from old drains, or fever patients, all go to the top of a building, end if there is no outlet it must stop there and endanger the health of persons occupying it. By leaving one room vacant, a window in it could be continually open and no one would suffer from bad air. A skylight in the roof would answer the same purpose, but these are scarcely ever opened.

WHOOPING-COUGH

Frequently when whooping-cough intervenes during the time of teething, the irritation of the o-ums somewhat abates. Some children have whooping-cough and diarrhea for some length of time, and upon recovery, show quite a number of teeth. I am not all in favor of encouraging any increased discharge from the bowels, but sometimes in congestive whooping-cough a little looseness is beneficial. Cholera often sets in just as the teeth have begun to break through the gums. The treatment, however, should be the same as if not teething. Great caution should be observed not to administer drugs containing laudanum; for by so doing, air and mucus collect in the air or bronchial tubes, inducing a stoppage in the breathing. Possibly suffocation and death have resulted from this cause in numbers of cases. Whoopingcough, if gently treated, seldom, if ever, proves fatal. I have had patients under my charge with it from four weeks old, upwards. It would, nevertheless, be well to keep the tender infant from exposure to whooping-cough for a while. It does seem as if sooner or later in life we are to encounter these peculiar complaints. The main thing to do to relieve the force of whooping-cough is to keep the chest and air-tubes warm, and, most of the time, moist. If there is danger of congestion, a warm poultice of flaxseed meal spread over the chest and throat, and keeping clear of dust, smoke, or smells of any kind, will aid much. By all means the nose should be kept running, which may be done by sweating the forehead and nose. Bronchitis or wheezing, like whooping-cough", is a disease that affects the air-tubes in a greater or less degree, the inflammation sometimes becoming very distressing. The treatment should be about the same as for whooping-cough.

PNEUMONIA

Pneumonia, which is lung fever, frequently sets in just about the time a child is getting teeth. When there is known to be inflammation of the sub-stances of the lungs, active treatment is called for. To the nurse, or mother, I will say that the surest signs of lung troubles are in the manner of breathing. If the nostrils flare at every attempt to take breath, or in other words, if they open and shut in quick succession, there is little doubt as to the presence of lung fever well advanced. Of course, there is great heat prostration and perceptible agony from pain, even in the infant of three or four weeks. Thousands of babes die annually from this disease, who have never looked out at a door or window; how is it? Quick breathing may be occasioned by extreme pain, but never flaring of the-nostrils without some lung pressure. Active measures to reduce the blood is the proper way to treat lung fever. The flaxseed meal poultice over the entire chest, or wrapping the body up in flannel cloths wrung out of hot water, and giving to drink, plentifully, of cream of tartar and gum-arabic water, – one teaspoonful of each dissolved in a pint of boiling water and a teaspoonful every hour to a child one month old, and upwards, increasing the quantity according to age, – all tend to reduce the fever.

Very young infants are liable to perish in the acute stage, yet where the constitution is solid, in older babes there is a chance, with proper, special treatment, of raising them. Patient watchfulness, pure air, and absolute quiet, in all such trying afflictions, will more than pay for the enduring.

SORE THROAT, OR TONSILLITIS

It is with the deepest regret that I have to say that, of late, nearly every case of inflamed or sore throat is termed "diphtheria" – a name which sends a severely depressing blow to the heart of any a true, devoted mother. It is a pity that simple, curable diseases should be given such long.

Technical names that parents get frightened out of all common judgment, and give up all hope of successful efTorts to save. I frequently hear mothers say, "I lost my boy just as I had entered him in school." And rehearsing the causes, they are invariably these! – teething, diphtheria, "pneumonia on the lungs," one or all; "He couldn't live," and explicit pains is taken to state that "the doctor said so." I will simply state here that the throat is very likely to be affected while getting the first four grinders, or at the age of from sixteen to twenty-four months; and the true condition of the membranes of the mouth and throat cannot be guessed at. They should be examined by a skilled practitioner, that the danger may be modified in the outset. An ordinary sore throat may easily be converted into a malignant type by improper treatment; as in case of the sore throat of scarlet fever, for instance, the greatest danger arises from giving hot drinks, or applying some severe irritant to the membranes of the throat. It is well in all cases of sore throat to apply cooling treatment; this may be done by the following means: Wring a cloth out of hot water, wrap it around the throat, and cover with a dry flannel. Change every hour or two; give plentifully of warm barley-water to drink. Anoint the glands of the throat and ears once a day with goose or fish oil (no camphor), aiming to keep the parts soft, thereby scattering the inflammation. The diet should be nourishing, as of scalded milk, or, if the bowels are dry, raw milk with oatmeal pudding. The throat and mouth should be swabbed out frequently with a weak solution of bread soda; also common salt is good to excite the glands on the back of the tongue, and assist Nature to carry off the disease. By these, and various other domestic means, the sequences of scarlatina, such as dimness of vision, deafness, and glandular knots, may be avoided. Severe physic should never be given a child if costive while teething. There are other methods which, if applied, will be more lasting in effect; such as wringing a flannel cloth out of hot water, and covering the bowels; giving a pretty warm bath once a day. If injections are given, great care should be observed not to injure the soft internal folds of the lower bowel, but they should never be used if avoidable. Repeated but small doses of Epsom salts, dissolved in warm sweetened water, are invaluable.

WORMS

Children who are allowed to eat candies, and unripe fruit of all sorts, are liable to be troubled with worms. Such children are constantly thirsty, and almost as constantly desiring to go to the water-closet. Young children that are fed on pure milk rarely have pin or stomach-worms; but the irreg ular slop-feeding of children gives great chance for their development. In nearly all cases where they are known to exist, a few grains of salt given in water early in the morning will drive them downward. Then three grains each of calcined magnesia and pulverized rhubarb, mixed in cold milk just moist enough to be drunk, should be given at bedtime. This continued for about one week, with solid food at regular hours, will drive them out of the system. If pin -worms appear in the back passage, the injections of salt water twice a week, and giving a teaspoonful of salt water to drink every morning, will generally give relief.

———

CHAPTER XIX.

GENERAL REMARKS

WE HAVE, no doubt, learned, through the histories of the past, that war, or any civil commotion, naturally interrupts the moral and physical condition of the people in whose midst it is carried on. Not far from a quarter of a century has elapsed since the close of our civil war, and really the moral and physical condition of some of the people, the more remote from the scenes of those terrible deprivations and conflicts, are just beginning to develop the worst consequences. It is my serious opinion that thousands of children die annually in the city of Boston, under five years of age, from diseases brought on through the excitement of expecting to go to school, the early change, the exposures from actual compulsory attendance, while the system has barely recovered from a lengthy prostration, and now needing fostering at home with regular meals and plenty of toys for amusement.

Many are the little children of three and a half, four and a half, and five years, that are still getting teeth, sent out in the streets to saunter along in the chill air of our hill-streets to some school-house. Heaven bless our schools, for they are invaluable; but may God change the minds of the people as to such early exposures, being best for the credit of our Commonwealth. In school at four and a half, and in the grave at five; or in school at five, and in some State Reform School at seven or eight! just when the mind is beginning to be formed. It is well known that diphtheria, pneumonia, and various contagious diseases are more prevalent where there has been some exciting cause. For instance, during the warm days at the breaking up of winter, when the snow is melting and the atmosphere is filled with vapors, one can see children of all ages wading about in running water, dragging sleds, moving snow; some heavily-clad feet well protected, while others are not supplied even with wraps, but with rubber boots, it may be, minus the toes. In a few days many deaths of this very class of children are reported in some locality or other. Children will sit or stand around in places injurious to the health, and will go into dangers where they seem really to be admired by some adults. In the hurry and excitement to go in the street, so much is lost of a chance to build a solid foundation either of health or character. I know it is hard to restrain little ones after they have tasted of so much freedom as is given them during the weakest period of childhood, the teething period. This is why I feel so anxious to do or say something that will assist parents to lighten their burdens in this matter. In the first place, let me advise, with all due feelings of respect, the entire abandonment of low, dark, bad-smelling, water-soaked basement kitchens to work in, and the adoption of a rule to live more on top of the ground, and less under the ground. The depression upon the system of any one who has been permitted to exercise in open daylight, is equal to that of being incarcerated. Some persons say they send children to school to get them out of the way; a child soon begins to know this, and gradually goes out of the way, until some aching tooth or biting pain sends him crying to his friend.

If rooms are occupied all on the same floor, it is much better for the health and comfort of all. Windows can be dropped from the top; or a swinging pane, set in the top of a sash, is a very good way to ventilate or let in fresh air. So few people that depend on their bodily strength from day to day, stop to think that pure air is the all-essential element, and that without light, air, and sun in their dwellings, the poisonous gases cannot leave them, but they must sooner or later succumb to them Children need a great amount of rest while growing. Yet few children are ever permitted to lay down during the day after entering the primary school. "Oh," said a mother, " children rest sitting in school." The probabilities are, that those little nerves are all on a stretch for the first six months (if they last that long). And they never rest except the meals are regular, the mind made happy, and the sleep quiet and sweet. Not only so; the nervous system of children is, in many instances, run down before entering school at all. Thus, through a desire to humor or cater to its seeming wants, a child is permitted to toddle about on foot, aided by some excitement, all day long, eat whatever it should not, fret and fume till it is literally outdone. This might be avoided by the exercise of a little early home rule, which could be the better understood by the time the child is old enough to enter a public school. If there are a dozen children in one family, each one should be supplied with a chair, according to its age; so that when the word is given to sit down, it may be understood a%3 obeyed. If children can conform to rules of order for strangers, they certainly will for their dear parents and guardians. Would it not be well for mothers and friends to withhold some of their indulgences from children who are entirely too young to appreciate their endearing acts, and bestow them more lavishly when the possibilities of experience will insure a reward? Would not a little more kind persuasion bring sunshine into the family circle? Would it not pay for every laboring man of a family to reserve an empty room at the top of the house for a playroom for his children? There is not the least doubt but that every mother would be made to rejoice from the advantage; if not at the top of the house, on the same floor with the sitting-room.

There is nothing particularly commendable in the habit of permitting cats and dogs to be closely imprisoned with children, as little ones are prone to put their mouths to everything; thus, there is a probability of worms making from the hair of such animals when swallowed. By the close observance of the different traits of mankind, I have been led to believe that true philanthropy is ingrafted into the human heart only through Divine agency. So that if belief in God and His attributes is entertained by each, no sacrifice will be considered too great for the sake of relieving the helpless ones within the family circle. Philanthropy cannot dwell in the heart of an eye servant, it must be inborn and unbiased in applications relative to human happiness. Too often, it happens that mothers give up all hope just at the weakest period in a child's life, willing, on the slightest pretext, to abandon the offspring of their body. Words are not adequate to. portray the lasting miseries that, in consequence, daily encircle the minds and bodies of the youth of our land. With many parents, the beginning to raise a family is novel and pleasing, but at the very time the most particular care is required, patience and watchfulness flag, so that it is no uncommon thing to hear mothers, in particular, declare their inability to rule and rear their own children. Would it not be well for mothers to make a little sacrifice for the sake of equipping the mind, that they may be able to dispense the required rudiments of moral and intellectual education at home, till a child is at least seven years old? Let mothers awake to duty; let them seek to know the causes of so many bleeding hearts and weeping eyes, and learn to compare effect with means, and means with ends; then the pall that is ever ready to obscure their sky of cheer, will rapidly disappear. We find, when comparing the statistical reports of the death-rates of children under one year old, that they are largest in those cities where the influx of immigration is constant, and the women, either from choice or necessity, are so engaged in other pursuits, that they do not take care of their young. Also that the death-rate of children under six years old, is greater in those cities where early home discipline is thwarted and early school privileges are the rule. But a few months ago, a gentleman informed me that he had lost his only daughter." What caused her death?" I inquired. "The doctor said she studied too hard; she was taken with a hemorrhage, and died in a short time." "Was she old enough to go to school?" I asked. "Oh, yes," was the answer. "She was five years and a half." I knew the child was delicate from birth, but, notwithstanding, her mother had taught her the alphabet at home. No wonder, the doctor said she "studied too hard."

The "mind your own business" policy goes down too well with some women, for when the doctor pronounces the sickness of their babe a hopeless case, they seem at once to give up all hope, they have no alternative, they are mute, and will not so much as direct a petition to Almighty God, the great Physician for relief. Would it not strengthen the advocacy of equal suffrage in a population of over three hundred and sixty thousand, if every woman would cultivate a desire to know more about the prevention of disease and the preservation of health?

Diminutive, sickly, halfdependent people, care little what party governs, so long as they, themselves, barely exist. By real, earnest, devoted measures, women may be enabled, within the next decade, to exercise the right of franchise, and fill positions of honor outside of the domestic circle. But the women that compose the domestic circle have been, are, and ever will be in the majority; these are the women that have the greatest work of reform before them, namely, that of nourishing in infancy, ruling in childhood, and persuading in youth, the children of their fireside, that their sons may not graduate from the highest school of State penitentiaries, nor the bright future of their daughters be blasted by reason of early abandonment to the mercy of State charities. Parents should hold on to their children, and children should stand by their parents until the last strand of the silken cord is broken. It is natural to the childhood days to sport and play. All cannot bear the early and long-continued expectations through adverse circumstances and frequent unpleasantness of a finale. The vexations of youth from these causes, often serve, no doubt, to embitter the mind against further progress. We need in every community educated men, it is true, but the foundation dependence is in healthy, moral men and women.

Children should not be asked if they like such and such things to eat, with the privilege of choosing that which will give no nourishment to the blood. You may as well ask a child if the new shoes hurt the feet, if it is advanced enough to know that the old ones must be continued till the new ones are changed. Too much is expected of little children for their own good. All of the bones of our bodies, when broken, will unite again; but if the enamel of the teeth gets cracked or broken off, they soon decay, and -will be destroyed if not cared for by the means of art. From the age of seven months to twenty years, man is being supplied with those thirty -two pearly bones with which to prepare the food for entrance into the stomach, that it may be converted into milk, from which blood, the life principle, is derived each day.

Headache and toothache, one or both, render the school days of many a youth burdensome. This, too, may be caused as much from cold feet, indigestion, and constipation, as from either arduous studies or decaying teeth. Some parents would stand in amaze if their sons or daughters were discovered perusing some work upon the anatomy and the preservation of the human teeth in youth; while the same parents would boast of the almost frenzied determination of their children to read every available love-novel; that, too, while the new teeth are daily pushing against decaying ones. The study of the science of Dentistry is wise and commendable to all. Pauperism, like familiarity, "breeds contempt"; therefore persons should try with all their mind and might to avoid its conditions. Is it too much for me to say that the excuse for a mother's consigning her child to some almshouse, while she goes free, can be but shallow? Unfortunately, the "I can't" finds many prompters, and gains the precedence in many instances, where renewed and determined resolution only is required to succeed in caring for the helpless, and governing the passions of the youth, until they are old enough to hire out, or be put to some trade. To labor is honorable. Mothers, before you forget the tie which binds you to your child, and deliberately consign it to the care of strangers, look into those dear little eyes. Remember, few ever return, or are restored, as was Joseph of old.

> Cast me not off, dear mother,
> Oh, cast me not off, is my plea,
> I have ears with which to catch the sounds
> Of rejoicing or murmur from thee.
>
> I've a look that ne'er has been given,
> Which can only be given to thee;
> I've a word that has never been spoken.
> But yet can be spoken so free.
>
> Yes, a token of gratitude ever
> Shall dwell on my lips for thee;
> I've a tear that has never yet glistened,
> That some day may trickle for thee.

In the bleak and changeable climate of Massachusetts, in the city and vicinity of Boston, for instance, there reside many families whose ancestors were born in a more genial clime. Therefore, it is not natural that they, themselves, should be able to endure exposures to hard fare, even had they been early accustomed to it in a warm, native clime.

Our women work hard, seemingly, and many of them against a heavy tide; nor does there ever seem to be an end to their toils. Especially do some of the laboring women of my race appear to work under heavy disadvantages; if the family is small, they are never through with their work; if it is large, there is a double excuse for having no time to rest; yet many real needful things are left undone. I have often wondered if such housekeepers, whose own affairs are neglected, and in whose homes things go to waste, while they take so much upon them of other people's work, never thought of the story of "filling a hogshead at the spigot that had no stopper at the bung."

So with our men who labor hard; they are anxious to keep the wolf from the door, and they thoughtlessly rise in the morning, go to work, perhaps, without breakfast, working for hours in a condition for odors, contagious or otherwise, to affect the system. Thus the liabilities to colds in the vital organs, which may go on for years, gradually undermining the general health, or may, as frequently happens, develop in lung fever, and consequent shattered constitution. The laboring men of my race, generally speaking, take much better care of the horses intrusted to their care than they do of their own health. Were men just as particular about what they themselves eat and drink, and how they dress and sleep, the deaths of young men of thirty and forty years would not be so common. Those who are not careful of their health die early in this climate, and their offspring *die earlier.*

It is not the blood we wish to keep hot, as some desire to do; this induces disease and premature decay. It is the body that needs to be kept warm while the blood is normal, or rather cool. This is just as easily done with man as with the horse.

Frequent baths, wearing all-wool flannels next the skin in winter, changing for thinner ones in hot weather, eating coarse dry food, taking less medicine, desisting from the use of tobacco and "firewater," – all tend to lengthen the days of mankind on this beautiful earth. It is authoritatively stated that the colored population decreases in Boston, but it is not all the fault of the climate; for there have been native Africans who lived to a great age here. It is the neglect, in a great measure, to guard against the' changes of the weather.

By seeking to get in possession of the comforts of life, and buying a little home, our men can yet be enabled to live, and raise up children who shall be an honor to that noble race with which we are identified, in point of strength and longevity. The Lord gave the qualities, it is for us to preserve and improve them for His final acceptance. Our Heavenly Father has provided a healing balm for every disease that man is liable to, and I am prepared to say that all diseases can be cured without the use of alcoholic stimulants. We have access to a large and varied field of remedies, both in the vegetable and mineral kingdoms, the virtues of which unfold to man in proportion to his possession of heavenly virtues.

Let me, in conclusion, appeal once more to the united efforts of mothers and fathers. Do not try to be blind when you are not. Can you not cut short the certain destruction that awaits your sons and daughters, through the influence of impressions gained by the constant perusal of fictitious, and, in many cases, corrupt library books? Will it not pay to prohibit those under age, or at least under fourteen, from reading even Sunday-School story-papers? We are aware many of them are given for the moral to be derived, but not more than one boy or girl in a hundred ever cares a fig for the moral.

Does any one believe that the majority of the little children who witness the farce of " Punch and Judy" on Boston Common every summer, gain a moral, or feel that it is wrong to imitate beating a wife, killing a baby, or hanging a black man? The popular adage, "No nigger, no fun," is why such schools are tolerated on our Public Parks. Are they not a curse to our land? May not such shameful scenes prove to be the primary lessons in pugilism, murder, and suicide? Possibly they best serve to prolong the barbarous system of flogging, whether it be by lashing to a post and applying the cat-o'-nine-tails, or otherwise. Then will it not pay to endeavor to cultivate inborn morals early in life, thereby shutting out a desire for vulgar and debasing sports? –

Volumes might be written in which could be inserted plans, which, if enforced, could not fail to prevent the adversities of life, the gloomy foreshadowings and prolonged deficiencies in health. Some do not wish to know about the human system, others cannot read, and more have no time to read, or think how to live and be happy; seeming to forget that our Heavenly Parent gave the earth, with all it contains, for man's inheritance. Many such are laboring day and night, and trying to educate their children, yet do not always turn the abilities of their children to good account. Books on the laws of health from the proper source could never injure the mind and morals; but would, if read aloud in the family circle half as often as trashy novels are thumbed over, prove a blessing more lasting than gold. Let us strive to know more about ourselves, – it is human, it is Christianlike to do so. Then will there be minds from which to select students for the college, that maycome forth to the community graduates in Pharmacy, Surgery, Dentistry and Medicine. It is well known that many noble-minded women have graced the chambers of the sick with good service, in different conditions of need, too; but at the present, women appear to shrink from any responsibilities demanding patience and sacrifice, or rather seem not to rely on the union of their strength with that of our great Creator, in time of need.

What we need to day in every community, is, not a shrinking or flagging of womanly usefulness in this field of labor, but renewed and courageous readiness to do when and wherever duty calls.

———

PART SECOND.

MISCELLANEOUS INFORMATION

ALL THE OBJECTS in the material world are divided into organic and inorganic. The principle of life is always associated with organic bodies, examples of which are animals and plants. Quite a number of inorganic substances go to make up the human body, – to wit: Water, air, lime, magnesia, iron, potassium, sulphur, sodium, phosphorous, and many more.

HUMAN LIFE

Through the aid of scientific researches, we are informed that the development of a being begins with a soft jelly-like substance. Later, the parts intended for bone, become cartilage or gristle, progressing with more or less uniformity from a few hours after conception, till about the seventh month of pregnancy.

Anatomists nearly agree in stating that not more than six of the bones are ossified at birth, the greater number being finished at different periods of childhood. The lower portion of the vertebrae or backbone is not usually completed until after the twenty-first year of adult life. The bony framework of the adult man or woman is composed of about 246 bones, including the teeth. These are covered by about twice that number of muscles or fleshy supports. The muscles, cords and ligaments, which serve as so many bands for the support and protection of the body, are generally much larger and firmer in men than in women. The custom of suspending wearing apparel from the shoulders, conforms to the laws of nature; as those muscles are so arranged as to admit of considerable pressure without injury. Pressure upon the soft parts, as tying many bands around the waist, or tight lacing, is apt to cramp the internal organs of digestion, and crowd them out of their natural position, thereby inducing headache, or other unpleasant feelings.

WOMANHOOD

Begins with the appearance of the monthly sickness, at which times all undue exercise of the body should be avoided. Disobedience to the rules of decorum and the laws of health at such times, may induce ovarian inflammation, dropsy, consumption, and even barrenness.

It is a great mistake to administer brandy, gin, or any alcoholic or narcotic stimulant to girls for the relief of pain, when the periods are coming on. Opiates may destroy the functions, while alcoholic drugs can only relieve by blunting the sense of feeling, through the deceptive influence of intoxication.

Hot water foments, applied perseveringly, will bring more certain and permanent relief.

Menstruation begins much earlier in some girls than in others, yet is natural from the 11th to the 18th year, depending upon the state of the health, also, climate.

MORAL RESTRAINTS

An enema should never be given to infants in the presence of older children Little girls have been lacerated, and thus injured for life, through accidents growing out of imitating mother, or "playing sick," and giving injections. A young girl should be subject to the advice and protection of her mother or guardian, till sufficiently able to care for herself. Poverty, with chastity, is an enviable condition.

INTERNAL ORGANS OF WOMAN

The internal organs consists of the heart, lungs, liver, stomach, spleen, kidneys, bladder, intestines, or guts; the uterus, or womb, and ovaries, or eggs.

The heart is in the centre of the breast, pointing toward the left nipple; the lungs are on each side; the stomach lies below the true ribs, in the left side; the liver, with the gall-bladder attached, is situated below the true ribs, on the right side, reaching across toward the left side.

The spleen, a spongy melt-like viscus, is attached to the stomach and liver somewhat, but situated under the left side of the stomach; the kidneys are situated on each side of the spine or backbone, just above the waist; the bladder, into which the urine drops, is situated in front, just below the umbilicus, or navel; the uterus, or womb, is situated just behind the bladder; the ovaries are situated on each side, and a little behind the womb. Their office appears to be to secrete the menstrual flow, and also to supply whatever is needful in the formation of a new being. The womb is to receive and protect the impregnated germ, together with the vessels through which it is nourished from the mother, till the ninth month, or time of labor, at which time it is dangerous to drink stimulants unless directed by a physician.

The large intestine arises on the right side of the abdomen, extends up and across in front, just above the navel, then descends, terminating in the rectum, or straight outlet, just behind the womb.

In case of dry colic in men and the aged, rubbing with the hand, and steaming with hot cloths over the right side and down the spine, will sometimes induce an operation of the bowels when other means have failed. Blood, in all animals, is the life fluid; in man it is obtained through the mastication and digestion of his daily food and pure air. The blood is considered to be pure when we feel well, that is, can eat with pleasure, pursue vocations of livelihood, and enjoy refreshing sleep, but impure when the reverse. Physic can act beneficial only by hunting out and removing the obstructions to a natural flow of the digestive juices; but it does not, nor cannot purify blood. Blood medicines is a name used in reference to those which are employed to supply a principle wanting in the blood, but they do not make blood. Therefore, blood is supplied, and can be maintained without the intervention of art. There is scarcely a principle natural to the blood, but that can be obtained from something upon which we daily subsist.

A person may have pure blood, and yet suffer from obstruction in its circulation.

INFLAMMATION OF THE OVARIES

The ovaries are liable to affections from cold; the most frequent of which is acute or dumb aching pains, accompanied with great heat, depression of spirits, and thirst. It often seizes one while sweeping, or otherwise exercising. It not unfrequently comes on while asleep in bed, having the character of cramp, particularly after having wet or cold feet, as it is through the feet such sensations travel rapidly to those organs.

Treatment. – A pad made of hops or any soothing herbs, wet in hot vinegar, and laid over the lower part of the bowels and over the kidneys. Internally, one and a half teaspoonfuls of Epsom salts, and one-eighth as much of pulverized cinnamon, dissolved in a little warm sweetened water, observing absolute quiet, will, in most cases, give speedy relief. Opiate treatment should always be left to the discretion of a physician. It is the collections from repeated attacks of ovarian inflammation that give rise to tumors. They, too, can be cured if taken in time, but it requires total abstinence from all kinds of fish or stimulating food, or drinks, and very regular bowels.

RHEUMATISM

Rheumatism, or nerve pain, of which there are several characters, is nevertheless caused by taking cold, in some certain condition of the system, at almost any time of life. Persons who get in cold or damp beds, or sleep in cold, ill-ventilated rooms without night-clothes, or otherwise neglect to comfortably prepare the body for the maintenance of pure blood, are mostly liable to rheumatism in some form. It may last for a few days only, then again, it may remain in the system for years. It frequently attacks one part of the body and goes off, leaving a lasting depression, remote from the seat of the attack. Ofttimes it affects the nerves that control the organs of voice and speech; more especially in those persons who use tobacco and "toddy."

Treatment. – In nearly all cases, in full habits, having been exposed to great heat, alternating with cold, purging, sweating and extreme quiet, will relieve. Anointing the parts with warm goose-oil, or boiled olive-oil, is highly serviceable. In cases of long standing, with poor blood, the opposite treatment is indicated, *i e.*, food or medicines that create warmth, and supply principles wanting in the blood; such, for instance, as beefjuice, rare-done beef-steak, lamb chop, corn bread, pure wheat bread, milk, and stewed fruits.

Articular rheumatism, or that affecting the joints, long after the acute or first attack, can generally be cured by feeding the joints, as it were, from without. Ligaments and joints are not quickly affected by what enters the circulation, but very much can be gained by wrapping the joints with bandage, wet in some stimulating sedative of which hot water takes first rank, pulverized opium and water next. Dissolve ten grains in as much hot water as it will require to wet the bandages, apply and cover with a dry flannel. Liniments should be used with caution, as they tend to close up the pores of the skin.

Very much may be gained by taking a hot salt bath twice a week, not necessarily going to the sea-side. In all cases of rheumatism, with feelings of languor or loss of appetite, a tea of seneca snake root and valerian is advisable, and may be drank at pleasure, cold. Also, a cold infusion of hoarhound and hops, made sweet with maple sugar, is good, if continued for quite a while. Dose – a pint during the day.

SOFT BONES

Soft bones, or a tendency to crooked limbs, in many families, may arise from a taint of ill-humors, or rachitis in the parents, or even grand-parents; likewise, weak joints. The preventive means are, not to keep the infant too hot, or closely bound, while asleep. Children born free from any imperfection may develop distorted, if allowed to creep around or sit on a cold or damp floor, be tossed into a bed between cold sheets, when the nerves are excited and the blood is warm. It would require but little outlay to provide close flannel drawers for children to creep around in; besides, the nation would be blessed, in the future, with men and women possessing firm muscles, with well-fed marrow in their bones.

Treatment. – Wholesome food, frequent warm salt baths, comfortable clothing, sufficient sleep, and that in a comfortable place. HEAD-ACHE so frequently complained of by both sexes, generally denotes some irregularity, either in the manner of eating or sleeping. For instance, strong tea is binding in nature, but there are persons who "must have it," yet, nevertheless, are usually constipated or nervous. Eating a lunch just before retiring will mostly insure headache, as will, also, over-taxation of the mind or body.

HEMORRHOIDS

Hemorrhoids, or Piles, may be brought on by whatever irritates the folds of the rectum or back passage; as sudden cold, frequent attempts at stool with dry bowels; frequent and severe physicking, or the passage of fecal matter rendered acrid by the indulgence in highly-seasoned food, alcoholic drinks, or late suppers.

Cure. – Abstinence from heating food or medicines, bathing the lower portion of the spine with warm water, applying simple goose -oil, or the simplest ointment, whether the sores extend to the opening or not. The patient should take, as a cooling potion, a teaspoonful of Epsom salts in warm water, two or three times a week. Nothing reduces the blood in the parts more speedily; and there is not the least danger, as is erroneously sup-posed by many, of taking cold by its use. There is a thousand times more danger in numerous other drugs and potions given under the cover of a great name, to cure the piles.

It is an error to suppose that certain remedies are only serviceable at certain times and in certain places, at certain times of the year. Every means possible should be put forth to reduce the piles before submitting to an operation; a thing that is seldom needed, but nevertheless is frequently done.

LEUCORRHOEA, OR WHITES

This is a very common complaint among women of all ages and conditions of life; but not more so, probably, than seminal weakness in men, – a similar complaint, by the way. It frequently comes from taking cold, after fatigue, which may run its course with some degree of fever, languor and chill; during which time ulcers may form on the membranes of the vagina, or entrance to the womb. These ulcers may remain quite a while, and cause a continuance of the discharge, or they may come off, and leave weak patches, even in virgins. This complaint is not contagious, but if allowed to remain about the parts, may become offensive and excoriating. It requires much the same treatment as catarrh; hence frequently receives the name, catarrh of the womb. It may come from getting up too soon after confinement.

Treatment. – If ulcers are known to have formed, they should be removed in the surest manner, that the introduction of the speculum may be dispensed with as soon as possible. After their removal in that way, the cure can be accomplished sooner, but ulcers can be removed without the introduction of the speculum in very small women. If the evidence is conclusive that ulcers have formed, the remedy for their removal can be applied with less pain and displeasure with the vaginal syringe. No astringent washes, such as alum, oak, bark, or lead, are in place while fleers remain. When there is no unhealthy discharge from the vagina, there can be no need of using a syringe. Salt sea or home baths, nourishing food and rest; applying a wet bandage, warm, during the hours of rest, and keeping the bowels free without the use of severe physic; avoiding laborious work for a while, will give great relief.

The constant use of preparations of iron is binding; and while, at the same time, they may tone up the muscular fibre, they may but invite a renewal of the discharges, by reason of pressure upon the vaginal walls from the loaded rectum. It is a complaint which may at any time give rise to evil imaginations, therefore should be cured as soon as possible. It has been thought, that using the treadle sewing-machines has increased the liabilities to leucorrhoea; but I have yet to conclude whether it is from the use of the machines or the manner in which they are used by most women.

In the first place, the operator sits too far from the machine, thereby causing a motion of the whole body, while she leans too much forward; secondly, operates too fast; thirdly, works too long at a time; fourthly, allows herself but little time to eat or sleep. And, what is more than all, frequently gets angry with the machine, unstrings it, and gets it in as bad condition as she has her own nerves.

I would suggest, that weakly women use a sewing machine that is turned by hand. Whatever causes a discharge, should be speedily removed, as the first means of cure.

FALLING OF THE WOMB

Numbers of women persist in saying their womb is down; I must admit that there are many who suffer from a partial prolapsus, or protrusion of the mouth of the womb; the causes of which are usually traceable to hasty deliveries, miscarriages, overlifting, pressure from a distended bladder, or constipated bowels. But the most frequent cause of a bearing down or a dragging sensation, is from weakness of the whole muscular system. The walls of the canal that leads to the womb, partakes largely of this weakness, which of course is increased by the retention of urine or fecal accumulations in the lower bowels.

There are a variety of uterine difficulties that afflict women of all classes and conditions of life. Yet it is somewhat encouraging to know that the cure of each is possible when rightly understood.

Treatment. – If the bowels are kept free by taking a teaspoonful of Epsom salts, dissolved in warm water, about three times a week, bathing frequently, and absolute rest observed, relief will be certain.

A pessary or ring should never be worn if avoidable. There are other means to resort to less unpleasant and more certain to give permanent relief. All misplacements of the womb should be rectified at once.

CHANGE OF LIFE

The appearance of the menses in girls, denotes the beginning of womanhood; but the irregularities which the periods sometimes exhibit from the ages of 35 to 50, have given rise to the term " change of life."

Women are considered to be in their prime at from 25 to 45, and if careful of habit, may escape any perceptible irregularity save but a few months before the entire cessation, or till after the fiftieth year of their age.

What is needful for a pleasant and healthy cessation of the turns, is a more strict observance of the rules of self-preservation. In some cases, where the menses appear early, they leave early.

Climate and the state of the mind, and general health, very often influences the periodical flow; the mere change of residence for a few hundred miles, causing them to vary or disappear entirely, even in young girls. It is a great mistake for young women, thus affected, to seek a doctor or doctress who is considered an expert in " bringing the turns on again." Probably any amount of mischief has been done by neglecting to cultivate patience in this matter.

In the decline of life, the cares become burdensome, and the system is in a more irritable condition, therefore liable to cold. The ovaries sometimes become enlarged, causing the abdomen to bloat, and sometimes present the appearance of dropsy, or tumor; or a general enlargement may take place. There may be periodical flooding of bright or dark, even black blood, and large pieces of clot may cause great pain for days, then pass away unattended by any serious change in the general health.

Very many women begin to notice the change by feelings of suffocation, flashes as of hot steam, alternating with a slight chilly feeling. If at any time perspiration is free, it should be encouraged rather than suppressed. It is better to endure the hot feelings and save the lungs, than to expose them by inhaling cold air through the tubes, or driving the perspiration in on to them. Fanning, rushing into cold air, drinking ice-water, all tends to throw the danger internally, inducing paralysis. When the feeling of suffocation comes on, it is decidedly best to sit quiet. When there is much fluttering of the heart, it is a good plan to take one or two swallows of cool water, just as it is coming on; this sometimes has the effect to retard it for weeks.

Treatment – Avoid over-heated rooms or exciting scenes; keep the bowels free without severe physic. Use coarse plain food, drink very little of fluids, avoid spices, stimulants, and secure cheerful exercise for the mind, with an abundance of outdoor scenery; cultivate a love for the gifts of our Heavenly Father, seek to do good for those who are worse off than yourself, and all will come out right.

After the turns have ceased altogether, a woman may live to a good old age, and fill many hours of usefulness to her sex.

Should the beats of the heart interrupt sleep very much, it is a good plan to drink about a half-pint of hop tea, sweetened with brown or maple sugar, at bed-time.

If the heart beats full and heavy, three grains of Bromide of Potassium should be dissolved in cinnamon water, and drunk at noon and night, for a week at the time, then left off to watch the result; and continued, if needful. When there is great heat of the skin without perspiration, a little mustard should be added to the daily baths for a while. Much depends upon keeping the blood in a normal state at such times, and if the luxuries of life are indulged in, the tendency is to fire the blood, so to speak.

Meats, and sweets, or pastries, induce thirst, simply by their chemical combination with the juices of the stomach; and the more water is drunk to quench the thirst, the longer will the distress continue.

It is not at all improbable that the frequent sudden deaths of women about the age of 36, is owing to taking cold through some imprudence, at this time. Great care should be taken not to have the beatings of the heart stopped too suddenly.

All women are not affected alike; many never experience any heart trouble, whilst a great number are subject to it from early maiden life. If there is much wind in the bowels, it is a good plan to take about five grains of pulverized magnesia and three of pulverized cinnamon, in a little sugar and water, every morning; it gives a gentle operation, and may be repeated at will.

Irregularities of the menses, like the event of pregnancy, very frequently occasions cramp in the stomach, for which many women boast of drinking gin, or some equally volatile stimulant; this should never be done. Putting on cloths wrung out of hot water, and sipping hot water with a little mustard in it, will soon relieve. In case of pregnancy, the cramps mostly cease with delivery.

CATARRH - COLD IN THE HEAD

Catarrh is caused by exposure of the face and glands of the neck to sudden draught, while the blood is quite warm. The mucus that drops from the internal membranes of the head becomes dry, accumulates in flakes, pieces of which gradually drop down on the soft palate and organs of the voice, thus obstructing the air-passages. If it is permitted to go on, it is apt to cause inflammation of the bronchial tubes.

Northeast, and easterly winds, favor its development much, but, with timely aid, it may be cured.

BRONCHITIS, OR INFLAMMATION OF THE AIR TUBES WHICH LEAD TO THE LUNGS

Treatment. – In all cases of catarrh or bronchitis, means should be used to soften the glands and muscles of the neck. Warm steam should be applied to the nostrils and inhaled into the lungs. Medicines taken into the stomach, cannot reach the difficulty. Much may be gained by snuffing a little warm salt water up through the nostrils. When there is great distress from mucus in the air-tubes, about three grains of pulverized ipecac should be added to about a gill of hot water, and the steam inhaled into the lungs. All inhalants should be boiling hot, and used repeatedly for an hour or more. Inhaling cold air after sitting in a close atmosphere, will induce an attack of bronchial inflammation, or thickening of the air-tubes, in persons of all classes and conditions. Persons who are liable to frequent attacks of bronchitis, are apt to imagine that their lungs are affected, since it prevents a free use of the voice in singing or speaking audibly. I will repeat that this complaint generally terminates with a loss of tone in the lung substance, caused by the failure of the tubes to supply them with oxygen or air; notwithstanding, one may live on for years with it. Sudden changes of air, food or medicines that contract or depress muscular or nervous vitality, may cause suffocation and death at any moment.

When there is much cough present in chronic cases, inhalations of tar, pine bark, or roasted coffee, are beneficial. I never derived any benefit from the use of preparations containing camphor, in the treatment of diseases of the air passages; but have always succeeded with remedies that moisten, soothe, and warm.

BURNS AND SCALDS

For ordinary burns or scalds, cover the parts well with molasses, and give some internally. If blisters have not formed, this will prevent them; and if they have formed, the water should be let out, and the molasses well applied. It will keep out the air most effectually, and draw out the fire in a short time. Also, chilblains, skin or scalp sores, either on infants or adults. Corns, tetter, etc., may be cured by covering the parts at night with molasses, and washing it off in the morning with a weak solution of borax. In scalp sores of infants a little sweet oil should be added to the molasses.

CORNS, OR CALLOUS

Corns, or callous, whether on the feet of children or adults, come from wearing shoes that are too short and too wide, or otherwise ill suited, the friction of which, when walking, creates festers, the matter of which dries and becomes a corn.

Treatment. – Remove the cause, keep the feet clean, and comfortably clad.

SORE THROAT

This term is generally applied to all forms of throat troubles; but the most frequent cause of difficulty in swallowing comes from cold attended with swelling, and some degree of inflammation of the tonsils, hence tonsillitis. The palate, or curtain like arrangement over the root of the tongue, usually partakes of the irritation. The uvula swells, or becomes inflamed, and rests on the root of the tongue, creating a disagreeable sensation in the attempt to swallow. The palate is then said to be "down," when, in fact, it is not down, but enlarged. Ulcers frequently form on the tonsils, or almond like glands, inducing extreme suffering for weeks, when it could be cured in a few days.

Treatment – Apply with a quill, or hair pencil, a grain or two of bread soda (carbonate of soda), and give one teaspoonful of Epsom salts dissolved in warm water daily; at the same time, keep the neck moist during hours of sleep by the application of cloths wrung out of hot water, until relief is obtained. Epsom salts should be of the finest quality, well dissolved, and sweetened with sugar, whenever administered. The quantity should be reduced or increased to suit the age and condition of the patient.

DIPHTHERIA

This disease is usually ushered in by complete lassitude or loss of strength. The patient appears to lose intelligence, has no disposition to fret or laugh, the nervous powers seem to be blunted, with complete loss of appetite.

The chances of recovery are more favorable when the disease is rightly understood in the onset. This can seldom be the case, especially among the indigent, for in those instances the true nature of the complaint is overlooked, till it is too late to change the course of the malady.

Treatment – Medicines and external baths tending to reduce and brighten the blood, are of great importance. Of the medicines, bromide of potassium, given in from three to four grain doses, or two drachms dissolved in four ounces of water, given by tablespoonful doses three or four times a day for an adult. If the body is kept wrapped in a wet blanket, and changed every twenty-four hours, having it warm when first applied, it will greatly assist the recovery. Every means possible should be employed to keep the throat open. As this dreadful disease appears to arise from cold, irritation, and poisons in the blood, affecting the whole system, it may be a question if whiskey and such stimulants are beneficial in the first stage. Stimulants may be employed throughout the disease externally with great satisfaction, alternating with water baths, for if they are going to revive the powers at all, they will do so more readily and permanently by absorption from without.

As yet the treatment of diphtheria appears to be undecided by the medical faculty; an ailment must be well understood to insure decided treatment.

SCROFULOUS OR GLANDULAR SWELLINGS

may develop by exposure to sudden atmospherical changes, but all glandular enlargements are not a sign of scrofulous taint.

Nearly all of the ordinary swellings of the neck, or of any of the glands, may be entirely removed by the continued application of salt moistened with the pulp of apple. Hot salt-water baths are scattering, as is also an occasional anointing with the ointment of helebore.

Should they fill out with pus, they should be carefully lanced and the matter encouraged to flow out by applications of warm water or a poultice of flaxseed meal; should it not run freely and appear firm, add a little honey over the surface of the poultice for a short time. When the wounds are healthy they may be healed over by the application of an ointment prepared by melting white pine resin and tallow together. The system must be kept open, and the blood well fed at the same time, as poor living both propagates the disease and retards its cure. Scrofula frequently terminates in consumption.

TUMOR. FALSE GROWTHS

May develop in or on any part of the body, in either sex; but in women, most likely to form in the uterine regions. Some of the principal causes have been mentioned in Part I. I will here advise the general management: – Avoid eating fish, eggs, oysters, pork, vegetables of a gaseous nature, or any stimulant drinks; also avoid anything that may depress or excite the mind. As much of the distress which frequently accompanies tumor is the result of wind and loaded bowels, it is best to keep them free by small but repeated doses of warm Epsom salts; frequent hot salt-water baths; anointing the entire body with ointment of helebore, or goose oil. The dress should be of comfortable material. Where there is much bloating, a decoction of water, pepper herb and horse radish root, maybe drank at will for months; likewise, hop sweetened with brown sugar induces sleep. In this way one may live on comfortably for years with tumor.

BRAIN FEVER

In all cases where it is known there is a tendency of the blood to the head, the patient should be placed in a cool, quiet room. The hair should be shaved, or closely cut off; cloths wrung out of warm water may be kept continually over the scalp and back part of the neck. The feet and ankles as well as the wrists should also be kept moist during the height of the fever. Small doses of Epsom salts, say one quarter of a teaspoonful, dissolved in a little warm sweetened water, to a child from one to five years old, will generally relieve the blood-vessels, if given long enough to produce large passages from the bowels. The same remedy should be increased for adults. Also the bromide of potassium, administered as in case of diphtheria, is excellent.

It is usually some irregularity, over-work, or undue excitement, some way or other, that induces the alarming symptoms of brain fever.

But, at all events, it shows that there is an overcharged condition of the blood vessels, which should be promptly relieved. Efforts to this end should be both general and special. I have here inserted the general course, which is to reduce the blood in density by keeping the system open. Applications of ice, or ice-cold baths, over the head, after the fever is at its height, does not always prove beneficial to the general circulation. Ice may cause the blood to congeal in the parts, and thus prevent a chance for the removal of the pressure, through the ascending and descending blood-vessels. Cold water checks the flow of blood, while, on the other hand, warm water assists it to flow. It is just this assistance that is needed to free the system from all poisonous irritants, and when timely and rightly applied it cannot fail to relieve.

FORMULA FOR MAKING DOCTRESS CRUMPLER'S VEGETABLE ALTERATIVE

Take of fresh Indian posey and water pepper herbs, each one ounce; white pine bark, or tops, one half ounce; horehound herb, one fourth. Simmer in two quarts of water in a covered vessel four or five hours. Have three pints when strained; then add two and one-half pounds of loaf sugar. Boil briskly to a clear, thick syrup; pour out, and stir in while hot, one teaspoonful of pulverized mandrake root. Strain again through a fine cloth, and, when cold, bottle and keep in a cool, dark place. If podophyllin, the concentrated mandrake is used – which I prefer – only one half-teaspoonful is required to a quart of syrup. Dose for an adult, from one half to two thirds of a small wineglassful once a day while resting. Dose for small children, in case of bloating, worms, cough, from half to a whole teaspoonful at bedtime for a short while. Good to remove old colds from continued exposures, morbid craving for tobacco, alcoholic beverages or other blood poisoning idols, for which the dose is one teaspoonful in a glass of cold water at every inclination to drink, chew, or smoke.

Perseverance will insure success. No remedy should be continued after relief is obtained; too much physicking impoverishes the blood.

———

NOTE

IN THE PARAGRAPH on Sore Throat, page 102, I alluded to the danger of giving hot drinks in scarlet fever: the same precautions were intended for measles, or any of the skin diseases. But owing to a circumstance which occurred with a young mother since the publication, I am constrained to add some special advice for the management of measles. This disease usually appears in the latter part of winter or the first of spring. Children of various ages are liable to take it. This disease comes on with some degree of sick headache, hot, dry skin, and not unfrequently with cough and sore throat. A person may have it more than once, it may be carried around in the clothes of visitors, or retained for some time in the bedding, wall papers and carpets. It is very dangerous to give hot drinks, to hasten the pimples to appear; they usually do so about the fourth day after the fever begins, and if nothing was given, unless the person was kept very cold indeed, they would appear. It is this mistaken interference with Nature that causes many fatal terminations of measles. The severe headache, heat, swollen face and eyes, denote that the treatment should be rather cooling, in order to mitigate the suffering. As a general thing measles need not be considered to be any more than a cold; with a gentle purge, warm baths, and drinks of warm water and lemonade, the patient will be all right in about eight or ten days. But as the lungs are liable to be more or less affected, a physician should be called in, that their true condition may be known in the commencement.

ERRATA

On page 16, line 7, for mama, read *mamma*.

On page 50, line 21, for panacea read *panada*.